COPD - AN UPDATE IN PATHOGENESIS AND CLINICAL MANAGEMENT

Edited by **Cormac McCarthy**

COPD - An Update in Pathogenesis and Clinical Management
http://dx.doi.org/10.5772/intechopen.68194
Edited by Cormac McCarthy

Contributors

Patrick Geraghty, Wendy Ezegbunam, Prangthip Charoenpong, Khushboo Chokshi, David N Smith, Adrian Cargill, Lillian Chow, Kimberly Foley, Cristian Oancea, Emanuela Tudorache, Voicu Tudorache, Thomas Hering, Ipek Candemir, Rajneesh Malhotra, Outi Vaarala, Tim McDonnell, Michelle Casey, Cliona O'Donnell, Amy Mulkerns, Orla O'Carroll, Eamon Mullen, Joanna Peart, Conor Burke

Published by InTech
Janeza Trdine 9, 51000 Rijeka, Croatia

Publishing Process Manager Dajana Pemac
Technical Editor SPi Global
Cover InTech Design team

First published February, 2018
Printed in Croatia
Legal deposit, Croatia: National and University Library in Zagreb

Additional hard copies can be obtained from orders@intechopen.com

COPD - An Update in Pathogenesis and Clinical Management, Edited by Cormac McCarthy
p. cm.
Print ISBN 978-953-51-3782-5
Online ISBN 978-953-51-3783-2

For EU product safety concerns:
IN TECH d.o.o., Prolaz Marije Krucifikse Kozulić 3, 51000 Rijeka, Croatia,
info@intechopen.com or visit our website at intechopen.com.

Meet the editor

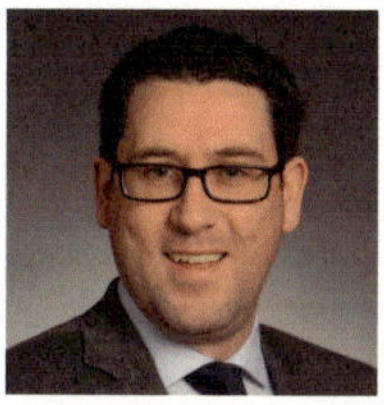

Cormac McCarthy, MD, PhD, MRCPI, is a scholar of rare pulmonary disease at the Cincinnati Children's Hospital and the University of Cincinnati Medical Center, Ohio, USA. He graduated from the Royal College of Surgeons in Ireland in 2007 and went on to complete training in internal medicine and pulmonary medicine at the Beaumont Hospital, Dublin, and the Royal College of Physicians of Ireland. He further completed a genetic pulmonary disease fellowship at the Cincinnati Children's Hospital and the University of Cincinnati Medical Center. His major research and clinical interests include rare and genetic lung diseases such as cystic fibrosis (CF), alpha-1 antitrypsin deficiency (AATD), pulmonary alveolar proteinosis (PAP), idiopathic pulmonary fibrosis (IPF), and lymphangioleiomyomatosis (LAM), among others.

Contents

Preface

Chronic obstructive pulmonary disease (COPD) is a major cause of morbidity and mortality worldwide and is estimated to become the third most common cause of death over the next decade. The knowledge of COPD pathogenesis and the disease course has greatly improved this progression in understanding and continues to have significant implications in the management of this condition. A more comprehensive awareness of the pathophysiology, underlying inflammatory processes, and multisystem comorbidities has led to advances in care and development of novel therapeutic agents.

Novel areas of interest in COPD pathogenesis include further development of animal models to investigate the pathways driving pathogenesis, a better understanding of the genetics and epigenetics of COPD, the role of the microbiome, and an increasing appreciation of many comorbidities associated with COPD and their effect on mortality and morbidity.

This book intends to provide the reader with a brief overview of these topics and also provide an in-depth review of the current nonpharmacological clinical approaches to managing patients with COPD.

Cormac McCarthy, MD, PhD,
Rare Pulmonary Disease Scholar,
Cincinnati Children's Hospital and University of Cincinnati Medical Center,
Ohio, USA

Section 1

COPD: Pathogenesis and Co-morbidities

Chapter 1

Animal Models of Chronic Obstructive Pulmonary Disease

Lillian Chow, David Smith, Khushboo Chokshi,
Wendy Ezegbunam, Prangthip Charoenpong,
Kimberly Foley, Adrian Cargill and Patrick Geraghty

Additional information is available at the end of the chapter

http://dx.doi.org/10.5772/intechopen.70262

Abstract

Chronic obstructive pulmonary disease (COPD) is the third leading cause of death in the USA and currently there are minimal therapies specific for the treatment of COPD. To advance our knowledge on COPD pathogenesis and develop new therapeutics, animal models are needed that represent key clinical and pathologic features of the human disease. The primary animal models utilized to study COPD rely on several factors associated with disease progression, i.e. genetic and epigenetic changes, environmental exposures and the microbial flora of the lungs. Here, a systematic approach was taken to summarize and evaluate the current animal models employed to study COPD pathogenesis, comorbidities and exacerbations. The strengths and limitations of these disease models are also delineated. The rodent COPD models have been extensively utilized but several studies have highlighted the potential of larger animals as an additional approach. Due to the inherent heterogeneity of COPD, the usefulness of certain animal models may be limiting but still represent helpful means to explore gene functional studies, testing new therapeutics and the exploring the significance of microbial floral changes. Therefore, interpreting the findings from animal models for the study of COPD represents a critical approach in deciding possible future human therapeutics.

Keywords: disease models, COPD, animal, cigarette smoke, lung remodeling, comorbidities, exacerbation

1. Introduction

Chronic obstructive pulmonary disease (COPD) is one of the major cause of morbidity and mortality worldwide and a significant economic and social burden worldwide [1, 2]. COPD is defined as a disease state characterized by airflow limitation that is not fully reversible, associated with an abnormal inflammatory response of the lungs to noxious particles or gases [3]. Airflow is limited by airway inflammation [4], loss of lung elasticity [5], lung tissue destruction [6] and the narrowing of small airways [7, 8]. Most pulmonologists believe that parenchymal destruction (emphysema) and small-airway obstruction (chronic bronchitis) are the most significant phenotypes of COPD, as they both contribute to airflow limitation [9]. Therefore, when designing models of disease these two phenotypes are crucial when interoperating data to clinical significance. Emphysema is further characterized by augmented inflammation, irreversible destruction of alveolar walls leading to airspace enlargement, loss of elastic recoil and hyperinflation [10]. Most COPD models investigate emphysema characteristics.

Cigarette smoke (CS) inhalation is the primary etiologic risk factor associated with COPD. The age-adjusted mortality for COPD has increased over the past three decades [11] highlighting the need for better therapies [12, 13], increased COPD research and enhanced utilization of research models. In the US, the CS prevalence is estimated to be 15–19% of the US population (age 18 or older) [14] and smoking will remain a major public health issue in the coming years. It is estimated that 16% of all 8th graders have tried smoking and 17% of high school students continue smoking beyond graduation [15]. The smoking prevalence globally remains high, with CS rates at 28% in China [16], 27% in Germany, and 36% in Russia [17, 18]. These statistics will ensure that this disease continues to be a major public health issue for the foreseeable future and CS-induced COPD will likely continue to rise over the next decades. Projects predict COPD to be the third leading cause of death globally by 2030 [19]. Beyond smoking cessation, very limited options currently exist for therapeutic intervention to halt COPD progression. The mechanistic basis underlying the pathogenesis of both emphysema and chronic bronchitis is very complex, involving a combination of recurrent inflammation, enhanced autophagy, oxidative stress, protease/antiprotease imbalance, tissue injury, repair and cell death [20]. These changes are all modulated by environmental exposures and host genetics [21]. Clinical studies demonstrate that all smokers experience a range of pulmonary inflammation but only 15–20% of smokers develop severe progressive emphysema [22]. This disparity underscores the importance of susceptibility factors, a subset of which are almost certainly controlled by host genetics in addition to environmental exposures. Chronic bronchitis is almost three times more frequently diagnosed compared to emphysema in the COPD population in the US but emphysema is associated with a greater frequency of patient deaths [23]. To this extent, new research approaches are required to advance our understanding of the key players involved in COPD development and to identify new therapeutics for future treatment of both emphysema and chronic bronchitis.

To better understand this complex disease, multiple research model approaches are need. Much of our current understanding of the normal functioning of the lung and mechanisms of lung disease comes from these studies utilizing animals. A model is defined as a simplified system that is accessible and easily manipulated. The natural course of COPD in humans can take decades. However, the ideal models of COPD would involve inexpensive species which could grow quickly and in which disease induction occurs over a short period of time while still mimicking the human condition. There are other factors that must be discussed as well when considering a model of COPD, such as sex, age, animal strain/background, exposure dosing and frequency which can all significantly impact on data interpretation. In this chapter, we will outline several animal models that have been used to study the biological processes believed to play major roles in the pathogenesis of COPD. Currently, the majority of COPD research is conducted in rodents. We will also discuss whether data obtained from rodents can shed light on COPD in humans.

2. Models of COPD

While cigarette consumption is the main risk factor for COPD, up to 10–15% of COPD cases are not related to CS exposure. Therefore, other factors can contribute to COPD initiation and progression, and multiple models are required to decipher the key mechanisms driving the disease. At this time, the majority of animal models for COPD research focus on emphysematous characteristics. Three major experimental approaches are commonly employed for the induction of emphysema-like symptoms in animals: elastase lung instillation, CS exposure and genetic manipulation. These three approaches are employed because CS is the primary etiologic risk factor associated with COPD and its comorbidities, an imbalance between elastase and anti-elastase activity results in enzymatic degradation of elastin and emphysema formation [24], and predisposing genetic factors are associated with COPD initiation and progression [25–27]. It is also known that CS has a major impact on elastase imbalance [28] and can also modulate gene expression [29]. Therefore, CS inhalation is the preferred approach and the following sections will outline these exposure models. Several other models of chronic bronchitis will also be discussed in addition to the emphysema models. The primary approaches to establish a model of COPD in animals is summarized in **Figure 1**.

2.1. Elastase model

In 1963, Laurell and Eriksson reported that patients deficient for α1-antitrypsin developed emphysema at an earlier time in life due to an abundance of elastase [30]. This discovery is the primary clinical observation that influenced the development of the elastase model of emphysema. In 1965, Gross et al. [31] developed the first animal model of protease-induced induction of emphysema in rats by instillation of the plant protease, papain, into the lung. Subsequently, numerous other proteases have been utilized to induce emphysema [32–35], including cathepsin B and proteinase 3. The most common protease utilized currently in animal models is elastase, primarily isolated from porcine. Porcine pancreatic elastase (PPE) is inexpensive and administration of PPE has been shown to induce features that resemble pan-acinar emphysema and lung damage throughout the organ. This approach has been utilized in many species of animals for several decades. The most frequently documented species, administration routes of PPE and exposure outcomes are summarized in **Table 1**, and will be discuss here in depth.

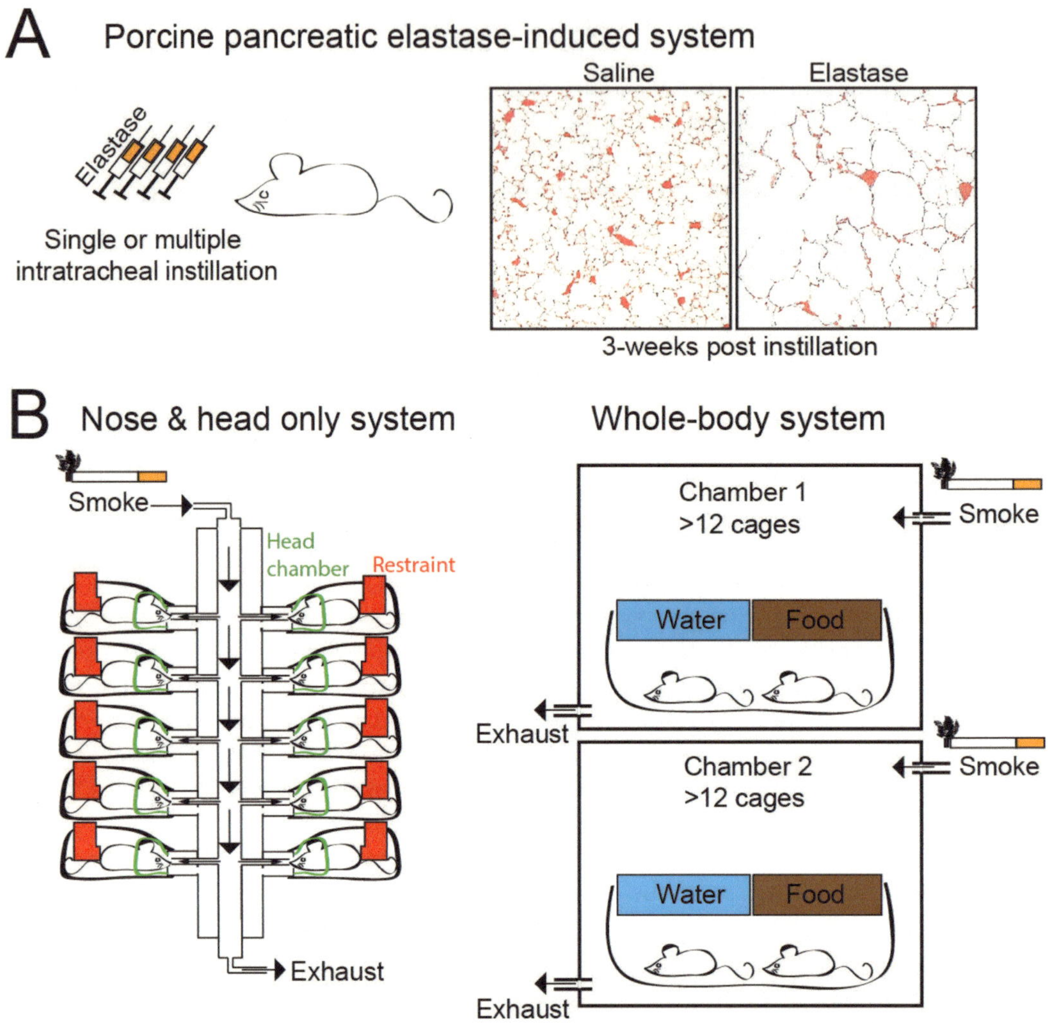

Figure 1. Typical mouse models for COPD. (A) Mice are administered a single or multiple intratracheal doses of PPE to induce an emphysema phenotype. One weeks onwards, there is significant evidence for airspace enlargements. Images show a typical profile following a single 1.2 Unit intranasal dose of PPE or saline and examination of the airways 3-weeks later by H&E staining. (B) A nose or head only (NHO) cigarette smoke exposure system requires animals to be restrained while they inhale the cigarette smoke. The whole-body system streams CS into a larger exposure system chamber and allows animals access to food and water without restraint.

As mentioned already, well-established genetic rodent background strains that utilize PPE-induced emphysema have been widely used as a model of COPD. Employing these strains/backgrounds, data from multiple studies are more reproducible and can be compared between groups. The animal genetic background is also critical for an appropriate control. Each strain has unique background alleles that may interact with and modify the expression of other genes upon establishment of a disease model or upon a stimulus, such as CS or elastase. Mice with different genetic backgrounds show disparate susceptibility to the development of

Animal	Reference	Strain	Administration	Outcomes
Mouse	[41, 44–49]	C57BL/6 and C57BL/6J	Intratracheal PPE	**Enhanced** airspace enlargements, lung volume and capacity, lung dendritic cells, MMPs, fibronectin degradation, epithelial cell apoptosis, alveolar epithelial damage, macrophages, neutrophils, lymphocytes, eosinophils, NK cells, CD8+ cells, A2M, HMOX1, MMP2, TIMP1, TNF-α, IL-1β, IL-4, IL-5, IL-6, IFN-γ and TGF-β. **Reduced** α1-antitrypsin, VEGF and DFCO
	[39, 41, 50]	BALB/c and BALB/cJ	Intratracheal PPE	**Enhanced** airspace enlargements, lung volume and capacity, compliance, hyperinflation, elastic and collagen fiber content, BALF hemoglobin content, M1 macrophages, neutrophils, lymphocytes, eosinophils, NK and NKT cells, CD4+ and CD8+ cells, NRF2, A2M, HMOX1, Arg1, Fizz1, MMP12, MMP2, TIMP1, SLPI, PrxI, HO-1, GST-Yc, NQO1, TNF-α, IL-1β, IL-4, IL-5, IL-6, IL-18, iNOS, IL-17A, IFN-γ and TGF-β. **Reduced** α1-antitrypsin, VEGF and DFCO
	[51, 52]	A/J	Endotracheal PPE	**Enhanced** airspace enlargements and lesions in the lung parenchyma distal to the terminal bronchioles
	[53, 54]	Swiss	Intratracheal PPE	**Enhanced** airspace enlargements, hyperinflation of the alveoli, alveolar collapse, MMP9 and TNF-α. **Reduced** VEGF and lung elastance
	[55, 56]	FVB/J	Intratracheal PPE	**Enhanced** airspace enlargements, lung volume, BALF hemoglobin content and alveolar surface area. **Increased** TGF-β, FGF-2 and GAG in BALF
Rat	[57–59]	Wistar	Intratracheal PPE	**Enhanced** airspace enlargements, NO release and leukocyte infiltration
	[60]	Sprague-Dawley	Intratracheal PPE	**Enhanced** airspace enlargements and increased dynamic compliance
Hamster	[61, 62]	–	Intratracheal PPE	**Increased** secretory cell metaplasia
Guinea pig	[63–65]	–	Intratracheal PPE	**Evidence** of interstitial edema, degradation of fibrous tissue, elastin degradation and enhanced alveolar enlargements. Loss of epithelial cilia and detachment of epithelial cells from the basement membrane. **Increase** tracheal hyperresponses to histamine, diaphragm fatigue, PMNs in tracheal submucosa blood vessels and infiltration of macrophages into the parenchyma

Animal	Reference	Strain	Administration	Outcomes
Rabbit	[62, 66, 67]	–	Intratracheal PPE	**Enhanced** airspace enlargements, apoptosis and 8-OHdG in lung tissues and reduced DLCO
	[68, 69]	New Zealand White	Endotracheal aerosolized PPE	**Enhanced** airspace enlargements, static compliance increase and decrease in expiratory flow and conductance
Pig	[70]	Yorkshire	PPE instilled into left lower lobe bronchus	**Evidence** of early edema, panlobular, centrilobular and paraseptal emphysema
Dog	[33, 71]	–	Endotracheal PPE	**Enhanced** airspace and septal destruction and enhanced airway enlargements
	[72]	Beagle	PPE injected through bronchi	Emphysema determined by chest computed tomography and histology
Sheep	[73–75]	–	Endotracheal and intrabronchial PPE	**Enhanced** lung resistance, bronchoconstriction and BALF levels of tissue kallikrein. **Decreased** tracheal mucus velocity

Abbreviations: GAG, glycosaminoglycan; NO, nitric oxide; PMNs, polymorphonuclear leukocytes; 8-OHdG, 8-hydroxy-deoxyguanosine; MMP, matrix metalloproteinases; NK, natural killer; IL, interleukin; TIMP, tissue inhibitor of metalloproteinases; TNF, tumor necrosis factor; IFN, interferon; TGF, transforming growth factor; NO, nitric oxide; SLPI, secretory leukocyte peptidase inhibitor; iNOS, nitric oxide synthases; VEGF, vascular endothelial growth factor; DLCO, diffusing capacity of the lungs for carbon monoxide; FGF, fibroblast growth factors; GAG, glycosaminoglycans.

Table 1. Animal models of COPD induced by elastase.

emphysema, when utilizing the elastase model of emphysema [36]. Globally, C56BL/6 mice are the primary background strain used to generate many types of genetically engineered mice, but they are one of many strains. Other strains, including BALB/c mice, are documented to be more sensitive to dose and time dependent to PPE injury, as demonstrated by significantly greater mortality, weight loss, decline in lung function, immune cell infiltration and loss of alveolar tissue [36]. This may be due to several genetic differences between strains. BALB/c and C57BL/6J mice have differing type 1 and type 2 cytokine-mediated inflammation responses that could play key roles in determining the resistance or susceptibility to many diseases. Altered allergy responses in subgroups of patients is frequently observed in COPD, frequently coinciding with eosinophilia and enhanced allergy responses or independent of allergies [37, 38]. Therefore, it is critical to select the appropriate mouse background when utilizing mice for COPD studies and the correct controls.

Most PPE-induced emphysema studies highlight the proteolytic activity of elastase on lung structural changes, such as higher airspace enlargements (measured by mean linear intercept) both in mice and in rats (**Table 1**). Furthermore, several studies report changes in extracellular matrix (ECM) composition, such as disorganized elastin, degradation of proteoglycans, and abnormal collagen remodeling [39]. However, these effects are dependent on several factors, including animal strain, PPE dose at each instillation, and number of PPE challenges. Mice subjected to repeat PPE administrations within 1-week developed a more severe phenotype, with enhanced alveolar destruction, weight loss, diaphragmatic dysfunction, exercise intolerance, and pulmonary arterial hypertension observed [40]. The pulmonary changes observed in PPE-induced emphysema in mice persisted for 6 months after injury induction [40] and therefore make this exposure model a useful tool in studying lung repair. Limjunyawong and colleagues [41] performed the most extensive study on PPE-induced emphysema in mice, utilizing two mouse strains, multiple doses of PPE over several weeks and extensive pulmonary function analysis. This study found strain, time and dose dependence on PPE-induced mortality, body weight loss, decline in lung function, lung inflammation and loss of alveolar tissue [41]. They also found heterogeneity in signaling associated with emphysema in each mouse strain.

Over the past few decades, other rodents have been utilized in models of PPE-induced COPD, such as rat, guinea pig, and hamster. These and other animal models are utilized as the mouse lung differs to human lungs in total lung capacity, left lung lobe number, lung pleural thickness, parenchyma percentage of the lung, alveoli size, blood-gas barrier thickness, trachea cartilage structure, number of respiratory bronchioles and airway generations, epithelium thickness and airway lumen size [42]. These other rodent models have several phenotypes that more closely reflect the human lung than the mouse. The lung volume and alveolar size have a closer resemblance to human lungs [42]. The airway of most rodents (except guinea pig) do not respond to leukotrienes, important mediators that cause bronchoconstriction in humans [43]. Depending on the species utilized, several confounding factors may not be functional in the model. Larger animal models of PPE-induced emphysema, utilizing rabbits, dogs, pigs and sheep, have observed enhanced airspace and septal destruction, and enhanced airway enlargements (see **Table 1**). Despite the many advantages of these larger species as an animal model of COPD, these species have not been widely used, probably due to limitations in terms of cost and reagent availability. Larger animal models do offer better understanding of lung structure than smaller animal models but most PPE-induced studies in these species were performed over 40 years ago, and the imaging and pulmonary function equipment was limited to address many parameters. Revisiting this approach in these species may be beneficial.

Overall, the intrapulmonary administration of tissue degrading enzymes, such as elastase, represents a useful approach to studying emphysema, especially when focusing on mechanisms to repair. PPE-based models are an attractive approach, since it is a simple exposure protocol with a single (or multiple) lung administration leading to significant and rapid changes. However, comparing this rapid method to the lifetime development of human COPD is very difficult since this method bypasses a large number of biological mediators. Equally, this method may reflect one subtype of emphysema and may not represent other sub groups of the disease. Therefore, the protease based models encompass several important features of human COPD but other methods, such as inhalation exposures, may also be required to better represent the phenotype of the human disease. The elastase model may be suited to tissue repair research.

2.2. Smoke exposure models

Like PPE-induced emphysema, a variety of animal species have been exposed to CS to mimic the human disease. Rodents (mice, rats, guinea pigs and hamsters) are the most commonly utilized species in CS exposure systems, but rabbits, ferrets, pigs, sheep and dogs have also been used (see **Table 2** for a summary of multiple studies). In parallel to PPE models, the severity of emphysema induced by the CS exposure model can be influenced by a variety of factors, such as differences in animal strains, smoke concentration, and duration of exposure, and the sex of the animal. The background strain of a mouse is an important factor in CS exposure with differing strains having varying susceptibilities or resistances to the development of CS-induced emphysema [76]. Smoke concentration measured in total particulate matter (TPM) per liter can also affect CS-induced emphysema development. Mice exposed to NHO CS inhalation, at concentrations of 75, 250, and 600 mg of TPM/L, show only a 13% increase in airspace enlargements (mean linear intercept) in animals exposed to 600 mg TPM/L after 28 weeks of exposure [77]. The TPM of mainstream CS is comprised of 4–9% of the total weight of cigarette smoke and is made up of many components, including polycyclic aromatic hydrocarbons, nitrosamines, phenol and nicotine. The TPM measurement excludes the gas and vapors in smoke. Therefore, regulated smoke concentration and the duration of CS exposure are critical steps in establishing a CS exposure model in animals. To prevent contrasting results when doing CS studies, Kentucky reference cigarettes (from the Center for Tobacco Reference Products) are used by many research groups throughout the world to aid in the standardization of the CS exposure model. Other species are very susceptible to CS-induced COPD, such as guinea pigs [78] and ferrets [79]. They develop COPD-like lesions and emphysema-like airspace enlargement within a few months of active CS exposure. By contrast, rat strains seem to be more resistant to the induction of emphysema-like lesions [80–83]. Equally, animal sex has been reported as a confounding factor in COPD susceptibility. One example are female A/J mice which develop emphysema 6 weeks earlier than their male counterparts [84].

Animal	Reference	Strain	Exposure	Outcomes
Mouse	[87, 89, 94]	C57BL/6	NHO	**Enhanced** lung hyperinflation, total lung capacity, compliance, alveolar enlargements, systolic blood pressure, circulating platelets and erythrocyte numbers, attenuate alveolar macrophage responses to inflammation, production of reactive oxygen species in heart and kidney and lipid peroxidation in heart, liver and kidneys. **Decreased** total nitric oxide plasma concentration
	[29, 109–113]	C57BL/6	Whole-body	**Enhanced** airspace enlargements, lung capacity, compliance, lung inflammation, serum TNF-α, vascular and myocyte dysfunction, TLR9 signaling, protease activity, lung cell apoptosis, and cytokine production. **Reduced** weight gain, muscle mass and type I and IIA oxidative fibers, lung tissue elastance, lung PTP1B activity, EPAS1 lung expression
	[90, 91]	BALB/c	NHO	**Increase** in oxidative stress in lung and heart, mitochondrial respiratory dysfunction, chronic inflammation, mucus hypersecretion, airway remodeling and emphysema. **Reduced** lung function
	[114, 115]	BALB/c	Whole-body	**Induced** lung neutrophilia, IL1α, IL1β and CXCL1
	[92, 93]	A/J	NHO	**Enhanced** susceptibility to tumorigenesis, hyperplasia, metaplasia, and inflammation of the nose and larynx and proliferative lesions of the lungs. **Delayed** cutaneous wound healing

Animal	Reference	Strain	Exposure	Outcomes
	[29, 116–118]	A/J	Whole-body	**Enhanced** airspace enlargement, right ventricle heart hypertrophy, lung cell apoptosis, infiltration of macrophages, neutrophils, lymphocytes, kinase activity, cytokine and protease expression. **Reduced** FEF50%/FVC, EPAS1 lung expression
	[115]	Swiss	Whole-body	**Enhanced** mast cell recruitment to cutaneous wound
	[119]	FVB/NJ	Whole-body	**Enhanced** airspace enlargements, immune cell recruitment to the lungs, RSV lung infection, lung cell apoptosis, BALF protein concentration, expression of S100A9 and MCP-1. **Reduced** PTP1B activity
	[120]	FVB	CSE IP injection	**Enhanced** airspace enlargements, prothymosin α expression, NFκB activity, MMP2 and MMP9
	[76, 121]	AKR/J	Whole-body	**Increased** inflammation, Th1 responses, macrophages, neutrophils, and T cells, oxidative stress levels in diaphragm and gastrocnemius. **Reduced** weight gain
Rat	[80–83]	Wistar	Whole-body	**Increased** gastric ghrelin, plasma TNF-α. **Reduced** food intake, weight gain, abdominal fat, plasma levels of leptin, insulin-like growth factor-1
	[122, 123]	Sprague-Dawley	Whole-body	Areas of blebbing and microvillus-like projections from the luminal surface, and micro-thrombi proximal to intercostal branches. **Enhanced** lung parenchymal destruction, pulmonary hypertension and pulmonary inflammation
Hamster	[5, 99]	–	Whole-body	**Induced** elevation of right ventricular systolic pressures, medial hypertrophy of pulmonary arterioles, lung chymase activity, Ang II levels and enhanced TGF-β1/Smad signaling. **Reduces** production of lysyl oxidase and the resynthesis of cross-linked elastin
Guinea pig	[97–99]	Hartley	Whole-body	**Increased** pulmonary artery pressure, right ventricle hypertrophy, raised respiratory resistance, airspace enlargement, intrapulmonary vessel remodeling, immune cell infiltration, CatK and CHOP expression, ERK and JNK phosphorylation. **Decreased** elastin and the loss of type III collagen in the alveolar walls
Ferret	[79]	*Mustela putorius furo*	NHO	**Increased** early-morning spontaneous coughs, sporadic infectious exacerbations, airway obstruction, goblet cell metaplasia/hyperplasia and mucus expression in small airways
Rabbit	[101–105]	New Zealand White	Whole-body	**Decreased** alveolar count, IRAK degradation. **Increased** ductal/destructive fraction, lung destruction, apoptosis, airspace enlargements, immune cell infiltration, intraparenchymal vascular congestion and thrombosis, intraparenchymal hemorrhage, respiratory epithelial proliferation, alveolar destruction, emphysematous changes and bronchoalveolar hemorrhage, lung and aorta expression of MMP1 and lung expression of TLR4

Animal	Reference	Strain	Exposure	Outcomes
Pig	[124]	–	Lungs only	**Enhanced** vasodilator response in the bronchial circulation, bronchodilatation and bronchial vasodilatation
Dog	[125]	Greyhounds	Whole-body	**Increased** parenchymal damage and inflammation
	[126, 127]	Beagle	Through a tracheostoma	Histological evidence of emphysema
Sheep	[128]	–	Unilateral inhalation	**Increased** gas exchange impairment and metabolic activity

Abbreviations: ERK, extracellular signal-regulated kinase, JNK, c-Jun N-terminal kinase; TLR, toll-like receptor; EPAS1, endothelial PAS domain protein 1; CXCL, chemokine (C-X-C motif) ligand; NFκB, nuclear factor kappa-light-chain-enhancer of activated B cells; FEF, forced expiratory flow; FVC, forced vital capacity; MCP1, monocyte chemoattractant protein-1; Th1, type 1 T helper; Smad, mothers against decapentaplegic homolog; Cat, cathepsin; CHOP, C/-EBP homologous protein.

Table 2. Animal models of COPD induced by cigarette smoke.

The experimental details of CS smoke and tobacco usage in humans are so varied that, currently, no single experimental CS exposure system can replicate the diversity of human smoking patterns. Therefore, CS models probably reflects only facets of COPD but they still represent the closest model of early human disease. In the following sections, we will outline the COPD models that utilize CS exposure. There are advantages and disadvantages with both types of CS exposure approaches, such as animal number, exact quantifiable exposure, exposure duration and end points of study. Additionally, a detailed breakdown of every published CS exposure publication up to 2013 is summarized by Leberl and colleagues [85].

2.2.1. *Nose or head only exposure*

The nose or head only (NHO) exposure model (sometimes referred to as mainstream CS exposure) was developed for the induction of COPD in animals that allows quantifiable concentrations administered to animals. Several species, including mice, are obligate nose breathers, which allows direct delivery of CS or aerosolized solutions to be delivered to the lungs. The NHO system requires restraining the animal so that their nose is inserted into a cone where they inhale the cigarette smoke [86]. During this exposure time animals are deprived of food and water. This method generates a uniform exposure that produces the desired emphysematous changes. However, the prolonged periods of restraint are stressful for the mice and the machine can usually accommodate only a limited number of mice (e.g. the Jaeger system has eighteen ports which is depicted in **Figure 1B**). NHO exposures are usually for short exposure times (30–60 min) and CS exposures are repeated several times daily [87]. The level of exposure can range from 75 to 600 mg TPM/m^3 [77, 87]. In animal research, TPM concentrations is typically a defining factor for characterizing whether a study is a passive or secondhand exposure model, in addition to a NHO or whole-body method. A recent study examining gene expression profiles in CS exposure models in mice compared to human cohorts demonstrated that low TPM induces genes mainly related to xenobiotic/detoxification responses, while higher TPM activated immune/inflammatory and xenobiotic/detoxification responses [88]. In the same study, one human cohort clustered closer to low TPM but another cohort clustered closer to a high TPM [88]. Therefore, certain biological features of the CS exposure model are dose dependent and may represent a critical factor in establishing a model.

There are multiple companies that manufacture NHO exposure systems, e.g. Scireq, CH Technologies, Buxco Research Systems, In-Tox Products and Promech Lab AB. NHO exposure machines are typically automated for unattended operation (delivery, lighting, positioning, and ejection of cigarettes). They control the CS puff volumes and rates, are adjustable for direct smoke or indirect CS exposures, and contain a sealed chamber that prevents smoke leakage. The machines are relatively compact in size. Typically, an animal is placed in an individual exposure tube, with a rubber seal around the animal's neck to minimize exposure to the head. The tube is mounted onto the exposure tower (see **Figure 1B**) and CS is applied to the system. Some exposure models are equipped with a pneumotachograph, to measure respiratory flow from movement of the animal's chest wall. Alternatively, these models can be modified to test potential new aerosolized therapies.

Similar to PPE-induced emphysema models, mice are the primary species utilized in CS exposure models. C57BL/6 mice are frequently utilized in NHO exposures [87, 89], but others have utilized BALB/c [90, 91] and A/J mice [92, 93]. NHO exposure to CS has been documented to result in increased lung hyperinflation, total lung capacity, compliance, alveolar enlargements, systolic blood pressure, circulating platelets and erythrocyte numbers. This exposure model attenuates alveolar macrophage responses to inflammation, production of reactive oxygen species in heart and kidney and lipid peroxidation in heart, liver and kidneys and reduced total nitric oxide plasma concentrations in C57BL/6 mice [87, 89, 94].

Gaschler and colleagues [89] report that NHO and whole body CS exposure systems attenuate innate immune responses in a comparable manner. However, some outcomes appear to be different between both exposures, with NHO smoke exposures failing to produce soleus muscle weight reduction [87]. TPM concentrations [88] and exposure duration may also be confounding factors leading to differences in these models. Several larger animal species are more susceptible to CS exposure and NHO exposure resulting in phenotype changes similar to the human disease. Ferrets have several similarities to human airway physiology and submucosal gland distribution. In a recent NHO chronic CS exposure model, ferrets demonstrated clinical features close to human COPD, such as early-morning spontaneous coughs, sporadic infectious exacerbations, airway obstruction, goblet cell metaplasia/hyperplasia and increased mucus expression in small airways [79]. Despite larger animals displaying a lung morphology closer to human, the mouse model is the favored model of NHO CS exposure induced COPD. However, new models like the ferret may be a better model to evaluate and characterize further in future studies.

2.2.2. *Whole-body exposure*

Whole-body systems (sometimes referred to as side-stream CS exposure) can expose animals to a mixture of both passive and mainstream smoke, released from the burning cigarette and puffed through the cigarette [95]. The passive and mainstream smoke streams are mixed and then propelled by a fan to a chamber containing the mice that are housed within their cages. The advantage of this system is that the mice freely move about and have access to food and water (**Figure 1B**). Thus, mice in this system can be exposed for longer periods of time daily. In addition, the whole-body exposure system allows for the exposure of large groups of mice. Some systems allow the exposure of greater than 120 mice simultaneously, enabling researchers to use large numbers of mice and to perform multiple experiments without stressing the animals beyond the CS exposure. There are several companies that manufacture whole-body exposure systems, e.g. Scireq and Teague Enterprises. These systems are also automated to help with ease of use.

Similar to the other COPD models already discussed, rodents are the most common species used in whole-body CS exposure models due to the wide variety of applicable gene expression manipulations. Several recent advances in pulmonary function testing in mice [96] will further enhance the usage of mice in CS exposure models. Other animal models include the guinea pig model, which has been shown to be susceptible to whole-body CS-exposures. CS exposure in guinea pigs induces several pulmonary and cardiovascular changes, such as pulmonary artery pressure, right ventricle hypertrophy, raised respiratory resistance, airspace enlargement, intrapulmonary vessel remodeling, loss of elastin and type III collagen in the alveolar walls, immune cell infiltration, protease and kinase activity [97–99]. Measurable emphysematous changes are also detected in rats following 2-months of whole body CS exposure [100]. Very few larger animals have been utilized in the whole-body exposure system, perhaps due to insufficient access to chambers large enough to contain these animals. Several studies have successfully exposed rabbits to whole body CS [101–105]. Mice do not produce MMP1, the major collagenase associated with COPD [106], but rabbits express MMP1 and its induction is CS triggered [103]. For the study of proteins not expressed in smaller animals or expressed at a different frequency to human, several larger animals may represent a better model option. Rabbits are relatively easy to handle and several transgenic animals are available [107], making them a good model for investigating lung-related diseases. Rabbits are also large enough to allow non-lethal monitoring of physiological changes during the course of the CS exposure but rabbits still have multiple differences in lung physiology to human [108]. Importantly, when deciding on a CS exposure model of emphysema, it must be noted that both NHO and whole-body exposure methods result in emphysema and other COPD symptoms in animals, and both represent good but not perfect models of COPD.

2.3. Genetic models of COPD

Prior to genome-wide association studies (GWAS) on COPD samples, several genes have been investigated in animals for susceptibility to COPD development and pathogenesis (**Table 3** is a summary from multiple mouse studies). GWAS and other genomic based studies have identified many further genes that are associated with COPD [26, 29] but functional studies are required to prove their importance in lung function and disease development. Currently, mice represent the most favored laboratory animal species to manipulate gene expression. The discovery of new gene manipulation approaches may alter this view, such as CRISPR-Cas9. CRISPR-Cas9 approaches in larger animals is an exciting new method for future COPD research. Several existing models will be briefly outlined here that alter susceptibility to environmental exposure

Reference	Mouse	Exposure	COPD susceptibility	Outcomes
[129]	*Itgb6*$^{-/-}$	–	Increased	**Spontaneous** development of age-related lung emphysema due to lack of ITGB6-TGF-β1 regulation of the MMP12 expression
[130]	Klotho$^{-/-}$	–	Increased	**Increased** aging, enlargement of the air spaces, destruction of the alveolar walls
[131]	Human *MMP1* expression	–	Increased	**Increased** disruption of the alveolar walls and coalescence of the alveolar spaces
[136]	*Mmp12*$^{-/-}$	CS	Resistant	**Reduced** smoke induced alveolar macrophage infiltration and emphysema
[139]	*Tnfr*$^{-/-}$	CS	Resistant	**Reduced** airspace enlargements and neutrophil infiltration
[138]	*iNOS*$^{-/-}$	CS	Resistant	Mice **protected** against emphysema and pulmonary hypertension
[143]	*Cd8*$^{-/-}$	CS	Resistant	**Blunted** inflammatory response and did not develop emphysema
[111]	*Tlr9*$^{-/-}$	CS	Resistant	**Protected** from smoke-induced airspace enlargements, loss of lung function, inflammation, protease activity, apoptosis, and inflammation
[144]	SOD1 overexpression	CS or elastase	Resistant	SOD1 **prevented** smoke or elastase induced airspace enlargements, neutrophil infiltration and lipid peroxidation product accumulation
[137]	*Cav1*$^{-/-}$	CS	Resistant	**Reduced** senescence of lung fibroblasts and pulmonary emphysema
[140]	*Mrp1*$^{-/-}$*Mdr1a*$^{-/-}$ *Mdr1b*$^{-/-}$	CS	Resistant	**Reduced** inflammatory and emphysema
[145]	*Il-18Ra*$^{-/-}$	CS	Partially protected	**Decreased** inflammation and emphysema
[144]	*Il-1R*$^{-/-}$	CS	Partially protected	**No induction** of inflammatory cell infiltration, small airway remodeling or matrix breakdown
[146]	Adiponectin$^{-/-}$	CS	Partially protected	**No induction** of inflammatory cell infiltration, airspace enlargements, tissue elastance or TNFα
[147]	SOD3 overexpression	CS or elastase	Partially protected	SOD3 **prevented** smoke or elastase induced airspace enlargement, impairment of lung function and exercise capacity
[148, 149]	*Il-17a*$^{-/-}$	CS	Partially protected	**Exacerbated** macrophage and $\gamma\delta$ T cells frequency, which trigger emphysema
[119]	*Ptp1b*$^{-/-}$	CS	Increased	**Enhanced** airspace enlargements, immune cell recruitment, apoptosis, and inflammation

Reference	Mouse	Exposure	COPD susceptibility	Outcomes
[132]	*Nrf2*$^{-/-}$	CS	Increased	**More** inflammation, oxidative stress, apoptosis and reduced antioxidants
[133, 134]	*Gpx1*$^{-/-}$	CS	Increased	**Enhanced** airspace enlargements, BALF neutrophils, macrophages, proteases, IL-17A, MIP1α, NFκB and AP1 activation. **Reduced** PP2A and PTP1B activity
[135]	*p53*$^{-/-}$	Elastase	Increased	**Increased** emphysema severity, macrophages, neutrophils, BALF CCL2, BALF TNF-α and lung oxidative stress

Abbreviations: ITGB6, Integrin Subunit Beta 6; SOD, superoxide dismutase; Cav1, caveolin 1; Mrp1, multi-drug resistance associated protein 1; Mdr1, multi-drug resistance gene 1; AP1, activator protein 1, CCL, chemokine (C-C motif) ligand.

Table 3. Gene modulated models of COPD in mice.

induced COPD or genetic alterations that result in spontaneous COPD development. There are two major approaches, i.e. gain-of function or loss-of-function. These gene manipulations can be targeted within the whole body or within specific tissue or cell types. Gain-of-function is achieved by gene overexpression in transgenic mice or expressing a human gene or variant of that gene. Alternatively, loss of function is achieved by specifically targeting loss of expression of a gene, by direct or chemical mutagenesis. The majority of studies performed in COPD utilize whole body knockout animals, where the gene was genetically manipulated in the embryo prior to development. Several genes have been linked with COPD since several knockout animals develop spontaneous COPD as they age, such as *Itgb6*$^{-/-}$ or klotho$^{-/-}$ mice [129, 130]. Equally, introducing a human gene into a mouse can result in COPD development without environmental exposures, such as lung expression of human *MMP1* in mice [131]. Most genetic manipulations require a "second-hit" to observe lung changes causing disease. Inducing a COPD phenotype by CS inhalation or PPE instillation in animals deficient for *Nrf2* [132], *Ptp1b* [119], *Gpx1* [133, 134] or *p53* [135] exaggerates COPD-like changes. However, most genetic manipulations have been associated with protecting against CS or PPE induced COPD, e.g. *Mmp12*$^{-/-}$ [136], *Cav1*$^{-/-}$ [137], *iNOS*$^{-/-}$ [138], *Tnfr*$^{-/-}$ [139] and *Mrp1*$^{-/-}$*Mdr1a*$^{-/-}$*Mdr1b*$^{-/-}$ [140] mice. Since COPD is an extremely complex heterogenous disease, many of these genes and others may all contribute to disease initiation and progression. The GWAS studies in humans have identified several other possible targets for future investigation, e.g. HHIP, CHRNA5, HTR4, FAM13A, RIN3, TGFB2, GSTCD-NPNT, CYP2A6, IL27-CCDC101, ADGRG6-GPR126, THSD4, ADAM19, TET2, CFDP1, AGER, ARMC2, RARB, EEFSEC, DSP, MTCL1, SFTPD, IREB2, HHIP, and FAM13A [141, 142]. The mouse model still remains the best species to manipulate gene expression in the lungs but new techniques will aid in larger animals being utilized in the coming years.

2.4. Models of bronchitis

As mentioned previously, the second phenotype in COPD is an airway model for chronic bronchitis. Several studies have focused on induction of bronchitis phenotypes in animals (see **Table 4** for a summary of several studies). Bronchitis models utilize noxious inhalants

Animal	Reference	Strain	Exposure	Outcomes
Mouse	[158]	BALB/c	SO_2	**Enhanced** neutrophilic inflammation, epithelial sloughing, ET-1 and TGFβ expression
	[154]	C57BL/6	NO_2	**Increased** airway (neutrophils and macrophages), goblet cell hyperplasia, collagen deposition in the lung parenchyma and airspace enlargements
Rat	[150, 151]	Sprague Dawley	SO_2	**Increased** pulmonary resistance, airway responsiveness to methacholine, immune cell infiltration (notably neutrophils), immune dysregulation, oxidative stress, mucin, accumulation of surfactant in lamellar bodies of alveolar type II cells, BALF levels of lactate dehydrogenase and N-acetyl glucosaminidase activity. **Reduced** dynamic compliance
	[159, 160]	Sprague Dawley	NO_2	**Increased** dopamine D(2) receptor expression
Ferret	[152]	*Mustela putorius furo*	SO_2	**Observation** of lesions with changes in ciliated cells, edema and cell infiltration. **Increased** coughing, nasal discharge and dried mucus
	[161]	*Mustela putorius furo*	NO_2	**Reduced** thoracic clearance function
Hamster	[160]	DSN	NO_2	**Moderate/severe** bronchiolitis and alveolitis development. **Increased** mitosis in Club cells and BALF surfactant

Animal	Reference	Strain	Exposure	Outcomes
Guinea pig	[162]	–	SO_2	**Increased** hyperresponsiveness to intravenously administered serotonin, degeneration, desquamation of epithelium, and edema of the lamina propria of the trachea and bronchi
	[163]	Hartley	NO_2	**Increased** BALF eosinophils and neutrophils, microvascular leakage in the trachea and main bronchi.
Rabbit	[164]	–	SO_2	**Increase** in sputum viscosity. **Decreased** respiratory rate and pO2 blood level
	[165]	–	NO_2	**Enhanced** destructive of walls and abnormal enlargement of the distal air spaces
Dog	[166]	–	SO_2	**Significant** ciliated cell damage
	[167]	–	NO_2	**Changes** in edema, congestion, interstitial irritation, bronchiolitis, and interstitial fibrosis

Abbreviation: ET-1, endothelin-1.

Table 4. Animal models of bronchitis.

such as sulfur dioxide (SO_2), nitrogen dioxide (NO_2), or ozone. SO_2 is a gaseous irritant which can be used to induce COPD-like lesions in animal models. Exposure to high concentrations of SO_2 daily results in chronic injury and repair of epithelial cells in rats [150, 151]. The exposure to high-levels of this gas ranging from 200 to 700 ppm for 4 to 8 weeks has been demonstrated to lead to neutrophilic inflammation, morphological signs of mucus production and mucus cell metaplasia and damage of ciliated epithelial in rats [150, 151] and ferrets [152]. Exposure of SO_2 to capsaicin-treated rats results in increased airway smooth muscle mass and increased airway responsiveness observed in these animals [153]. NO_2 is another gas that induces COPD-like lesions in a concentration, duration of exposure, and species susceptibility dependent manner [154]. Exposure to NO_2 (50–150 ppm) can reduce animal survival due to extensive pulmonary injury, including pulmonary edema, hemorrhage and pleural effusion. Sub lethal levels of NO_2 causes damage to cilia, hypertrophy of the bronchiolar epithelium and a type II pneumocyte hyperplasia in rats and hamsters [155, 156]. Mice exhibit similar lung responses to NO_2 exposure [154]. The administration of ozone [157] also causes significant lung injury with several features associated with human COPD. All three of these exposure models were utilized in several species of animals but are rarely utilized in current studies of COPD. A recent NHO chronic CS exposure model in ferrets demonstrated clinical features close to human bronchitis [79] and suggests that the animal species may be a deciding factor in bronchitis research. Overall, new approaches are needed to access bronchitis in animal models of COPD.

2.5. New models of COPD

Several novel models of COPD have been utilized recently, including investigation of biomass fuel and individual components of CS, i.e. nicotine. Several of these models will briefly be discussed in this section. One research group has developed a rapid COPD model in mice by daily injecting CS extract (CSE) into the abdominal peritoneal cavity [120, 168]. Airway enlargements and injury of cardiac and skeletal muscles are reported within 6 weeks of initiation [120, 168] but comparative studies to whole-body or NHO systems are required. Recent genetic analyses have identified $\alpha3$ and $\alpha5$ nicotine acetylcholine receptors (nAchR) as susceptibility loci for COPD [169]. The airway epithelium expresses $\alpha3$, $\alpha4$, $\alpha5$, $\alpha7$, $\alpha9$, $\beta2$ and $\beta4$ subunits for nAchRs [170], and their expression are highest on the apical cell surface, where exposure to inhaled nicotine occurs [171]. Several animal studies have already utilized nicotine in models of COPD, airway lung injury and tumorigenesis. CS from high-dose nicotine cigarettes induces more emphysematous changes than low-dose nicotine cigarettes in PPE pre-treated rats [172]. Nicotine enhances airway hyperreactivity in lipopolysaccharides (LPS)-challenged mice and inflammation in lung epithelial cells [173]. Nicotine also suppresses apoptosis in lung tumors [174].

These observations are important considering several new approaches for nicotine replacement therapy now being marketed, such as e-cigarettes. E-cigarettes are a relatively new product that has grown in popularity over recent years. E-cigarettes are devices that effectively deliver vaporized liquid nicotine to the lungs. The user can choose the nicotine concentration and devices can deliver a range of volumes. However, several additional studies have suggested that these products require further testing in animal models and human studies to evaluate short and long term effects. Recently, the US Surgeon General concluded that e-cigarette use among the younger population is now a significant public health concern [175]. The use of e-cigarettes enhances oxidative stress and inflammation in mice [176] and impairs immune defense against bacterial and viral infection [177]. Nicotine in e-cigarettes has also been implicated as the driving force of these changes in mice, with long-term inhalation of nicotine-containing e-cigarettes shown to increase airway hyperreactivity, distal airspace enlargement, mucin production, cytokine and protease expression [178]. There are some direct human disease correlations, with normal human bronchial epithelial (NHBE) cells grown at the air liquid interface exposed to nicotine-containing e-cigarette vapor showing impaired ciliary beat frequency, airway surface liquid volume, conductance of ion channels, decreased expression of genes associated with ciliogenesis and increased cytokine production [178]. The animal models used for these studies use either the e-cigarette device connected to a whole-body CS exposure model, outlined in section b.ii, or a whole-body nebulizer. Many companies have modified their NHO or whole-body exposure systems for e-cigarette research, which will expand on new animal models for lung research. Therefore, these models and others should be utilized in future studies of COPD and nicotine replacement therapy.

Models of air pollution have been used to examine several phenotypes of COPD, with exposures to diesel exhaust particulates (DEP) and other biomass fuels under scrutiny. Animals exposed to DEP daily via intratracheal instillation for 3-months have decreased IFN-γ levels in bronchoalveolar lavage (BAL) but elevated CD3+ T and CD8+ T cells increased in the lung parenchyma and airway enlargement [179]. Equally, exposure of mice to smoke or particles generated from dung [180] and wood biomass [181] have been associated with several parameters of COPD. These models used modified CS whole-body exposure systems. Studies like these are important as it is estimated that air pollutants and biomass smoke could contribute to over 4 million deaths annually in the developing world [182] and contribute to the 10–15% of COPD cases not related to CS exposure. Therefore, new models or modification of the current group of COPD models are required to identify new biological targets of COPD and potential new therapies for treatment.

3. Exacerbation models

Exacerbations are one of the most important outcomes for COPD patients, as they contribute to decreasing quality of life, loss of lung function, and increasing mortality and healthcare cost [183]. Modeling acute exacerbations of COPD (AECOPD) in animals is challenging due to the complex clinical manifestations. Most AECOPD are triggered by infection, usually viral [184] or bacterial [185]. This association of the presence of a microbial pathogen at the onset of AECOPD is the primary basis for the majority of AECOPD animal models. These models typically entail exposure of an animal, usually a mouse, to CS followed by infection with a virus or bacteria. Live pathogens can be difficult to work with and often require special containment facilities. Therefore, some groups have used purified components of the pathogen, such as lipopolysaccharides (LPS) [186, 187] or *Staphylococcus aureus* enterotoxin B (SEB) [188], or a stimulus that will mimic the immune response upon infection, such as polyinosinic:polycytidylic acid (poly(i:c)) [189, 190]. Several of these approaches and outcomes are summarized in **Table 5**. The most frequently used live pathogens utilized in AECOPD models are influenza [188, 191], rhinovirus [192], respiratory syncytial virus (RSV) [112, 119], *Streptococcus pneumoniae* [193] and non-typeable *Haemophilus influenzae* (NTHi) [193]. Most models utilize the CS exposure system, but several have favored the PPE method [192, 193]. The general consensus appears to be that the COPD status enhances the lungs susceptibility to infection, inflammation and worsens lung function in a similar manner to the human disease. A study by Foronjy and colleagues [112] infected mice multiple times with RSV during a chronic CS exposure to mimic repeat viral AECOPD observed in the human disease. Repeated

Animal	Reference	Pathogen	Exposure	Outcomes
Mouse	[188, 191]	Influenza	CS	**Enhanced** airway damage, inflammation and alters IL33 responses
	[192]	Rhinovirus	PPE	**Increased** airway inflammation, obstruction, goblet cell metaplasia, total lung volume and alveolar chord length. **Reduced** lung elastance
	[112, 119]	RSV	CS	**Increased** airspace enlargements, inflammation, cytokines, chemokines, protease activity, apoptosis and fibrotic areas. **Reduced** phosphatase activity
	[118]	Modified HIV	CS	**Reduced** $FEF_{50\%}/FVC$ and **enhanced** distal airspace enlargement, inflammation, apoptosis and protease activity
	[189, 190]	Poly(i:c)	CS	**Enhanced** pulmonary inflammation, airway hyper responsiveness, corticosteroid resistance, remodeling, apoptosis, fibrosis, TLR3 signaling, type I IFNs, IL-18, IL-12/IL-23 p40, IFN-γ, PKR activation and eIF2α
	[193]	Streptococcus pneumoniae	PPE	Increased mortality, inflammatory cells in BALF, and MMP-12, as well as enhanced emphysema progression
	[199, 200]	NTHi	CS	**Increased** pulmonary inflammation (MCP-1, -3, and -5, IP-10, and MIP-1γ)
	[186]	LPS	CS	**Enhanced** susceptibility to airway lung injury

Animal	Reference	Pathogen	Exposure	Outcomes
	[188]	SEB	CS	**Increased** BALF lymphocytes and neutrophils, CD8+ T lymphocytes and granulocytes in lung tissue, IL-13, CXCL13, CCL19 and goblet cell hyperplasia
Rat	[201]	NTHi	CS	**Increased** airway bacterial load, aggravated mucus hypersecretion and delayed mucociliary clearance
Guinea pig	[187]	LPS	CS	**Enhanced** airway resistance, lung volume, neutrophils, epithelial hyperplasia and emphysema

Abbreviations: eIF2α, eukaryotic initiation factor-2alpha; PKR, protein kinase; SEB, *Staphylococcus aureus* enterotoxin B; NTHi, non-typeable *Haemophilus influenzae.*

Table 5. Animal models of COPD exacerbations.

infection heightened airspace enlargements, inflammation, cytokines, chemokines, protease activity, apoptosis and fibrotic areas, while reducing lung phosphatase activity [112]. The same group recently infected mice systemically with chimeric HIV-1 virus that is capable of establishing chronic infection in immunocompetent mice [194] and exposed these mice to CS [118]. This altered HIV-1 infection enhanced CS-induced COPD features in the lungs of these mice and this new murine model can be utilized to study HIV-related COPD, which results in a heightened form of the disease in the HIV+ population [195–198]. Therefore, several animal models exist that can aid in our understanding of AECOPD.

4. Modeling COPD comorbidities in animals

COPD is frequently observed with comorbidities that directly affect patient's quality of life, increase the risk for exacerbations and increase rate of mortality [202]. There are many manifestations of COPD comorbidities, such as lung cancer, skeletal muscle wasting (cachexia), diaphragm muscle dysfunction, cardiovascular disease, osteoporosis and diabetes [202]. Several studies have suggested that a large proportion of COPD-associated deaths are attributed to comorbidities [203, 204]. Given that comorbidities have a significant impact on COPD patient survival and quality of life, researchers have utilized animal models to investigate systemic comorbidities associated with COPD. CS exposure models show extrapulmonary manifestations, similar to those frequently observed in COPD. Mice and rats exposed to CS have reduced body weight, fat mass, hind-limb skeletal muscles mass, grip strength and aerobic endurance [82, 205]. CS exposure also enhances pulmonary artery wall thickening, increased contractility and endothelial dysfunction in guinea pigs [99]. Chronic CS exposure was recently shown to alter several cardiovascular parameters, such as enlarging ventricular end systolic and diastolic diameters, reducing myocardial and cardiomyocyte contractile function, and disrupting intracellular Ca^{2+} homoeostasis, regulating fibrosis, apoptosis and mitochondrial damage [206]. Mice and guinea pig exposed to CS, displaying lung inflammation and emphysema, have pulmonary hypertension and significant impairments to right ventricular diastolic and systolic function and contractility [99, 207]. CS in mice also causes hypertension, endothelial dysfunction and cardiac remodeling [208]. Chronic CS exposure have also been documented to increase systolic blood pressure, circulating platelets and erythrocyte numbers, attenuate alveolar macrophage responses to inflammation, production of reactive oxygen species in heart and kidney and lipid peroxidation in heart, liver and kidneys in mice [94]. Multiple elastase instillations in mice leads to the development of pulmonary arterial hypertension [209]. Diaphragm muscle dysfunction can contribute to COPD comorbidity. Diaphragm fatigue and ROS production are observed in guinea pig PPE-induced emphysema [65] and mouse smoke-induced emphysema [121], which could contribute to this comorbidity. Enhanced susceptibility to tumorigenesis is also demonstrated in mice exposed to smoke [93]. The hamster inhalation model is the only model in which tumor induction by CS has been reproducibly achieved [210]. These combined changes would be predicted to contribute to multiple comorbidities in COPD patients. Research focusing on models of COPD comorbidities will greatly improve our understanding of key factors in loss of quality of life and mortality in the COPD patient population, and additional novel animal models investigating the link between COPD and comorbidities are needed.

5. Animal model limitations and what is missing in these models

Models of disease try to mimic the disease as closely as possible. Despite no disease model being perfect, many models are helpful tools in deciphering the pathogenesis of the disease. Regarding COPD and the models outlined here, all models yield several phenotypes of the disease. Each researcher must evaluate the outcomes they desire to observe and choose the appropriate model that best suits their needs. For example, most COPD models cannot reproduce the features of severe emphysema as observed in humans, i.e. GOLD stages 3 or 4. Most models, especially the mouse smoke model, only represent early COPD (i.e. similar to human GOLD stages 1 of COPD) regardless of exposure time. It is estimated that obstruction of 75% of the small airways is required before changes can be detected by routine pulmonary function tests (e.g. forced expiratory volume in 1 s (FEV1)) in humans [211]. The majority of morbidity and mortality occurs in COPD patients with severe disease [3]. This is a major challenge to undertake when developing a reliable model of COPD as this requires a considerable amount of time and enhances the frequency of animal death prior to testing the conditions of the model. If a severe stage of COPD is required for investigation, the PPE model may be the best model currently available to examine COPD. However, if researchers are examining disease initiation or progression the PPE model would not be ideal. Another challenge in animal research is in the measurement of lung function in very small mammals, such as mice. The use of the enhanced pause (Penh) in conscious mice as an indicator of airflow obstruction is not ideal and invasive methods remain more reliable. Several new technical advances have aided in enhancing the pulmonary function readouts in animals but further work is needed to correlate animal data to the human disease.

The many differences in lung morphology and physiology between humans and the animals utilized in research will definitely impact on data interpretation, such as mice being obligate nose breathers, having lower numbers of cilia, fewer Club cells, differences in airway mucus production and reduced submucosal glands in the trachea. However, the experimental approach must also undergo scrutiny. Studies do not define whether a new therapeutic treatment is started following disease initiation or in parallel with the disease triggering exposure (i.e. CS or PPE exposure). Many treatments may be useful in preventing disease initiation but will have little impact on the lungs following disease establishment. Several recent studies are now addressing this experimental problem but scientific reviewers need to assert this difference in studies. In mice, lung lesions and inflammation induced by CS inhalation do not progress after cessation of CS exposure but airway enlargements persist [212]. This may have a large impact on the methodological design of experiments in mice. Whether other species recover following CS exposure is unknown. Equally, new genetic targeted approaches should be employed after disease establishment. Genes associated with disease progression can be selectively knocked down or enhanced after disease initiation, rather than utilizing whole body knockout animals that may have lung disease phenotypes due to embryo development problems. Modifying current methodology in these ways will further aid in advancing current animal model data and interpretations. Future animal model COPD studies should assess the histopathological patterns of COPD and examine functional parameters of human COPD using imaging, airflow limitation, mucus hypersecretion, corticosteroid resistance, β-adrenergic bronchodilator responses, chronic cough and exacerbations.

Overall, several major factors limit the interpretation of data from animal models to the human disease. Many investigators expect the animal model to exactly mirror the human condition but COPD is a complex and heterogenous disease and the human disease requires further sub-characterization prior to designing animal models or interpreting current data from animal models. We must also remember that without disease models, the burden on patients would be vast to participate in clinical trials and donate samples. Equally, not utilizing animal models would only allow clinicians to undertake COPD research. Deciphering the key players of a disease requires multiple approaches from many research fields and animal models may have a significant impact on COPD treatment in a similar manner to oncology and cardiovascular research. There are many benefits in development and use of animal models of COPD, especially the understanding of the fundamentals of immune and inflammatory mechanisms. Clinicians will benefit from the input of animal researchers, immunologists, microbiologists, bioinformaticians and statisticians.

6. Conclusion

Current animal model technology allows researchers to investigate the mechanisms of airways dysfunction, the influence of genetics and the immunological factors that define physiological and signaling changes that drive COPD. There are numerous well-established exposure models of COPD that exhibit several characteristics of the human disease, but no model captures every phenotype of the human condition. Mice are the most common species utilized for COPD research as they are small in size, they have a fast gestation period, and cost of feeding and housing are far less than larger animals. Also, the mouse genome is extensively characterized and many genetically modifiable mice are available, as well as equipment and biological reagents designed specifically for mouse anatomy. It is far more cost effective to generate genetically manipulated mice than it is to do so in other species. Another advantage to the use of mouse models is that exposure to CS for 1 year represents approximately 50% of the animal's lifetime, thereby allowing a better representation of lifetime CS exposure. While there are many physiological differences between the mouse and human pulmonary systems, the mouse models of COPD represent good tools to further our understanding of the human disease.

Acknowledgements

Patrick Geraghty's research is currently supported by grants from the Flight Attendant Medical Research Institute and the Alpha-1 Foundation. The authors would like to also thank the Division of Pulmonary and Critical Care Medicine and Departments of Medicine and Cell Biology of SUNY Downstate Medical Center for their support, especially Dr. Robert Foronjy and Dr. Moro Salifu.

Author details

Lillian Chow, David Smith, Khushboo Chokshi, Wendy Ezegbunam,
Prangthip Charoenpong, Kimberly Foley, Adrian Cargill and Patrick Geraghty*

*Address all correspondence to: patrick.geraghty@downstate.edu

The State University of New York Health Science Center, Department of Medicine, SUNY Downstate, Brooklyn, New York, USA

References

[1] Murphy BS, Xu J, Kochanek KD. Deaths: Preliminary Data for 2010. N.V.S. Reports, Editor. Hyattsville, MD: National Center for Health Statistics; 2012

[2] Raherison C, Girodet PO. Epidemiology of COPD. European Respiratory Review. 2009;**18**(114):213-221

[3] Rabe KF, et al. Global strategy for the diagnosis, management, and prevention of chronic obstructive pulmonary disease: GOLD executive summary. American Journal of Respiratory and Critical Care Medicine. 2007;**176**(6):532-555

[4] Miller M, et al. Persistent airway inflammation and emphysema progression on CT scan in ex-smokers observed for 4 years. Chest. 2011;**139**(6):1380-1387

[5] Osman M, et al. Cigarette smoke impairs elastin resynthesis in lungs of hamsters with elastase-induced emphysema. The American Review of Respiratory Disease. 1985; **132**(3):640-643

[6] Coxson HO, et al. A quantification of the lung surface area in emphysema using computed tomography. American Journal of Respiratory and Critical Care Medicine. 1999;**159**(3):851-856

[7] Stewart JI, Criner GJ. The small airways in chronic obstructive pulmonary disease: Pathology and effects on disease progression and survival. Current Opinion in Pulmonary Medicine. 2013;**19**(2):109-115

[8] Hogg JC, et al. The nature of small-airway obstruction in chronic obstructive pulmonary disease. The New England Journal of Medicine. 2004;**350**(26):2645-2653

[9] McDonough JE, et al. Small-airway obstruction and emphysema in chronic obstructive pulmonary disease. The New England Journal of Medicine. 2011;**365**(17):1567-1575

[10] Snider GL. Chronic obstructive pulmonary disease: A definition and implications of structural determinants of airflow obstruction for epidemiology. The American Review of Respiratory Disease. 1989;**140**(3 Pt 2):S3-S8

[11] Miller N, et al. Trends in chronic obstructive pulmonary disease mortality. Missouri Medicine. 2000;**97**(3):87-90

[12] Hogg JC. A brief review of chronic obstructive pulmonary disease. Canadian Respiratory Journal. 2012;**19**(6):381-384

[13] Kim V, Criner GJ. Chronic bronchitis and chronic obstructive pulmonary disease. American Journal of Respiratory and Critical Care Medicine. 2013;**187**(3):228-237

[14] Schroeder SA, Koh HK. Tobacco control 50 years after the 1964 surgeon general's report. JAMA. 2014;**311**(2):141-143

[15] Arrazola RA, Dube SR, King BA. Tobacco product use among middle and high school students—United States, 2011 and 2012. MMWR. Morbidity and Mortality Weekly Report. 2013;**62**(45):893-897

[16] Li Q, Hsia J, Yang G. Prevalence of smoking in China in 2010. The New England Journal of Medicine. 2011;**364**(25):2469-2470

[17] WHO. Report on the Global Tobacco Epidemic, 2009: Implementing Smoke-Free Environments, in Tobacco Free Inititative. World Health Organization, WHO Press; 2009. pp. 1-136

[18] McCartney G, et al. Contribution of smoking-related and alcohol-related deaths to the gender gap in mortality: Evidence from 30 European countries. Tobacco Control. 2011;**20**(2):166-168

[19] Mathers CD, Loncar D. Projections of global mortality and burden of disease from 2002 to 2030. PLoS Medicine. 2006;**3**(11):e442

[20] Fischer BM, Pavlisko E, Voynow JA. Pathogenic triad in COPD: Oxidative stress, protease-antiprotease imbalance, and inflammation. International Journal of Chronic Obstructive Pulmonary Disease. 2011;**6**:413-421

[21] Yoshida T, Tuder RM. Pathobiology of cigarette smoke-induced chronic obstructive pulmonary disease. Physiological Reviews. 2007;**87**(3):1047-1082

[22] Kohansal R, et al. The natural history of chronic airflow obstruction revisited: An analysis of the Framingham offspring cohort. American Journal of Respiratory and Critical Care Medicine. 2009;**180**(1):3-10

[23] Statistics NCFH. Chronic Obstructive Pulmonary Disease (COPD) Includes: Chronic Bronchitis and Emphysema. Centers for Disease Control and Prevention. 2015. https://www.cdc.gov/nchs/fastats/copd.htm

[24] Snider GL. Experimental studies on emphysema and chronic bronchial injury. European Journal of Respiratory Diseases. Supplement. 1986;**146**:17-35

[25] Wilk JB. et al. Framingham Heart Study genome-wide association: Results for pulmonary function measures. BMC Medical Genomics. 2007;**8**(Suppl 1):S8

[26] Pillai SG, et al. A genome-wide association study in chronic obstructive pulmonary disease (COPD): Identification of two major susceptibility loci. PLoS Genetics. 2009;**5**(3):e1000421

[27] Wilk JB, et al. A genome-wide association study of pulmonary function measures in the Framingham Heart Study. PLoS Genetics. 2009;**5**(3):e1000429

[28] MacNee W. Pathogenesis of chronic obstructive pulmonary disease. Proceedings of the American Thoracic Society. 2005;**2**(4):258-266; discussion 290-1

[29] Yoo S, et al. Integrative analysis of DNA methylation and gene expression data identifies EPAS1 as a key regulator of COPD. PLoS Genetics. 2015;**11**(1):e1004898

[30] Laurell CB, Eriksson S. The electrophoretic a1-globulin pattern of serum in a1-antitrypsin deficiency. Scandinavian Journal of Clinical and Laboratory Investigation. 1963;**15**:132-140

[31] Gross P, et al. Experimental emphysema: Its production with papain in normal and silicotic rats. Archives of Environmental Health. 1965;**11**:50-58

[32] Janoff A. Elastases and emphysema. Current assessment of the protease-antiprotease hypothesis. The American Review of Respiratory Disease. 1985;**132**(2):417-433

[33] Janoff A. et al. Lung injury induced by leukocytic proteases. The American Journal of Pathology. 1979;**97**(1):111-136

[34] Lesser M, Padilla ML, Cardozo C. Induction of emphysema in hamsters by intra-tracheal instillation of cathepsin B. The American Review of Respiratory Disease. 1992;**145**(3):661-668

[35] Kao RC, et al. Proteinase 3. A distinct human polymorphonuclear leukocyte proteinase that produces emphysema in hamsters. The Journal of Clinical Investigation. 1988;**82**(6): 1963-1973

[36] Affairs, D.o.V. 2011 Survey of Veteran Enrollees' Health and Reliance Upon VA: With Selected Comparison to the 1999-2010 Surveys. Department of Veterans Affairs and Veterans Health Administration. 2012. https://www.va.gov/HEALTHPOLICYPLANNING/SOE 2011/SoE2011_Report.pdf

[37] Singh B, Arora S, Khanna V. Association of severity of COPD with IgE and interleukin-1 beta. Monaldi Archives for Chest Disease. 2010;**73**(2):86-87

[38] Singh D, et al. Eosinophilic inflammation in COPD: Prevalence and clinical characteristics. The European Respiratory Journal. 2014;**44**(6):1697-1700

[39] Padilha GA, et al. Therapeutic effects of LASSBio-596 in an elastase-induced mouse model of emphysema. Frontiers in Physiology. 2015;**6**:267

[40] Luthje L, et al. Exercise intolerance and systemic manifestations of pulmonary emphysema in a mouse model. Respiratory Research. 2009;**10**:7

[41] Limjunyawong N, et al. Experimental progressive emphysema in BALB/cJ mice as a model for chronic alveolar destruction in humans. American Journal of Physiology-Lung Cellular and Molecular Physiology. 2015;**309**(7):L662-L676

[42] Irvin CG, Bates JH. Measuring the lung function in the mouse: The challenge of size. Respiratory Research. 2003;**4**:4

[43] Drazen JM, et al. Comparative airway and vascular activities of leukotrienes C-1 and D in vivo and in vitro. Proceedings of the National Academy of Sciences of the United States of America. 1980;**77**(7):4354-4358

[44] Takahashi S, et al. Reversal of elastase-induced pulmonary emphysema and promotion of alveolar epithelial cell proliferation by simvastatin in mice. American Journal of Physiology - Lung Cellular and Molecular Physiology. 2008;**294**(5):L882-L890

[45] Harada H, et al. Upregulation of lung dendritic cell functions in elastase-induced emphysema. International Archives of Allergy and Immunology. 2009;**149**(Suppl 1):25-30

[46] Moreno JA, et al. High-density lipoproteins potentiate alpha1-antitrypsin therapy in elastase-induced pulmonary emphysema. American Journal of Respiratory Cell and Molecular Biology. 2014;**51**(4):536-549

[47] Hou HH, et al. Elastase induced lung epithelial cell apoptosis and emphysema through placenta growth factor. Cell Death & Disease. 2013;**4**:e793

[48] Ueno M, et al. Alendronate inhalation ameliorates elastase-induced pulmonary emphysema in mice by induction of apoptosis of alveolar macrophages. Nature Commu-nications. 2015;**6**:6332

[49] Cloonan SM, et al. Mitochondrial iron chelation ameliorates cigarette smoke-induced bronchitis and emphysema in mice. Nature Medicine. 2016;**22**(2):163-174

[50] Ishii Y, et al. Transcription factor Nrf2 plays a pivotal role in protection against elastase-induced pulmonary inflammation and emphysema. The Journal of Immunology. 2005;**175**(10):6968-6975

[51] Valentine R, et al. Morphological and biochemical features of elastase-induced emphysema in strain A/J mice. Toxicology and Applied Pharmacology. 1983;**68**(3):451-461

[52] Munoz-Barrutia A, et al. Quantification of lung damage in an elastase-induced mouse model of emphysema. International Journal of Biomedical Imaging. 2012;**2012**:734734

[53] Cheng SL, et al. Prevention of elastase-induced emphysema in placenta growth factor knock-out mice. Respiratory Research. 2009;**10**:115

[54] Santos LM, et al. Bronchial responsiveness in an elastase-induced mouse model of emphysema. Respiratory Physiology & Neurobiology. 2014;**194**:9-14

[55] Lucey EC, et al. Retinoic acid does not affect alveolar septation in adult FVB mice with elastase-induced emphysema. Respiration. 2003;**70**(2):200-205

[56] Buczek-Thomas JA, et al. Elastase mediates the release of growth factors from lung in vivo. American Journal of Respiratory Cell and Molecular Biology. 2004;**31**(3):344-350

[57] Furuya N, et al. Cell therapy with adipose tissue-derived stem/stromal cells for elastase-induced pulmonary emphysema in rats. Regenerative Medicine. 2012;**7**(4):503-512

[58] Bianchi A, et al. Three-dimensional accurate detection of lung emphysema in rats using ultra-short and zero echo time MRI. NMR in Biomedicine. 2015;**28**(11):1471-1479

[59] Boiati RF, et al. Evaluation of the anti-inflammatory activity of atorvastatin and its effect on alveolar diameter in a model of elastase-induced emphysema in rats. Drug Research (Stuttg). 2015;**65**(10):540-544

[60] Onclinx C, et al. Elastase-induced pulmonary emphysema in rats: Comparison of computed density and microscopic morphometry. Radiology. 2006;**241**(3):763-770

[61] Breuer R, et al. Proteolytic activity of human neutrophil elastase and porcine pancreatic trypsin causes bronchial secretory cell metaplasia in hamsters. Experimental Lung Research. 1985;**9**(1-2):167-175

[62] Lungarella G, et al. Effect of the novel synthetic protease inhibitor furoyl saccharin on elastase-induced emphysema in rabbits and hamsters. Experimental Lung Research. 1986;**11**(1):35-47

[63] Miyazaki N, et al. Ultrastructural studies of elastase-induced experimental emphysema. Japanese Journal of Experimental Medicine. 1979;**49**(4):241-250

[64] Willet KE, Mitchell HW. Effect of elastase instilled into the trachea on airways mechanics in guinea pigs. Pulmonary Pharmacology. 1988;**1**(3):139-152

[65] Tamaoki J. Effects of elastase-induced emphysema on histochemical properties of guinea pig diaphragm. Respiration. 1988;**54**(1):16-23

[66] Brenner M, et al. Effects of a novel implantable elastomer device for lung volume reduction surgery in a rabbit model of elastase-induced emphysema. Chest. 2002;**121**(1):201-209

[67] Baila B, et al. Tetomilast attenuates elastase-induced pulmonary emphysema through inhibition of oxidative stress in rabbits. Biological and Pharmaceutical Bulletin. 2012;**35**(4): 494-502

[68] Chen JC, et al. An animal model for lung volume reduction therapy of pulmonary emphysema. Journal of Investigative Surgery. 1998;**11**(2):129-137

[69] Nishi Y, et al. Elastase-induced changes in lung function: Relationship to morphometry and effect of drugs. Pulmonary Pharmacology & Therapeutics. 2003;**16**(4):221-229

[70] Noma S, et al. Sequential morphologic changes of elastase-induced pulmonary emphysema in pig lungs. Evaluation by high-resolution computed tomography. Investigative Radiology. 1991;**26**(5):446-453

[71] Woods JC, et al. Magnetization tagging decay to measure long-range (3)He diffusion in healthy and emphysematous canine lungs. Magnetic Resonance in Medicine. 2004;**51**(5):1002-1008

[72] Gotoh M, et al. Development of a canine model of pulmonary emphysema and imaging of the emphysematous lung with infrared thoracoscopy. Journal of Thoracic and Cardiovascular Surgery. 2003;**126**(6):1916-1921

[73] Scuri M, et al. Inhaled porcine pancreatic elastase causes bronchoconstriction via a bradykinin-mediated mechanism. Journal of Applied Physiology (Bethesda, Md.: 1985). 2000;**89**(4):1397-1402

[74] Susskind H. et al. Assessment of elastase-induced structural and functional changes in sheep lungs. Bulletin Européen de Physiopathologie Respiratoire. 1985;**21**(2):149-157

[75] Scuri M, Sabater JR, Abraham WM. Hyaluronan blocks porcine pancreatic elastase-induced mucociliary dysfunction in allergic sheep. Journal of Applied Physiology (Bethesda, Md.: 1985). 2007;**102**(6):2324-2331

[76] Guerassimov A. et al. The development of emphysema in cigarette smoke-exposed mice is strain dependent. American Journal of Respiratory and Critical Care Medicine. 2004;**170**(9):974-980

[77] Hodge-Bell KC, et al. Pulmonary inflammation in mice exposed to mainstream cigarette smoke. Inhalation Toxicology. 2007;**19**(4):361-376

[78] Wright JL, Churg A. Cigarette smoke causes physiologic and morphologic changes of emphysema in the guinea pig. The American Review of Respiratory Disease. 1990;**142**(6 Pt 1):1422-1428

[79] Raju SV, et al. A ferret model of COPD-related chronic bronchitis. JCI Insight. 2016;**1**(15): e87536

[80] Tomoda K, et al. Changes of ghrelin and leptin levels in plasma by cigarette smoke in rats. Journal of Toxicological Sciences. 2012;**37**(1):131-138

[81] Esquivel AL, et al. The effect of obesity and tobacco smoke exposure on inflammatory mediators and matrix metalloproteinases in rat model. Toxicology Mechanisms and Methods. 2014;**24**(9):633-643

[82] Kamiide Y, et al. Chronic exposure to cigarette smoke causes extrapulmonary abnormalities in rats. Environmental Toxicology and Pharmacology. 2015;**39**(2):864-870

[83] Gomita Y, et al. Effects of standard cigarette and nicotine-less cigarette smoke inhalings on nicorandil plasma levels in rats. Pharmacology. 1990;**40**(6):312-317

[84] March TH, et al. Modulators of cigarette smoke-induced pulmonary emphysema in A/J mice. Toxicological Sciences. 2006;**92**(2):545-559

[85] Leberl M, Kratzer A, Taraseviciene-Stewart L. Tobacco smoke induced COPD/emphysema in the animal model-are we all on the same page? Frontiers in Physiology. 2013;**4**:91

[86] Nemmar A, et al. Evaluation of the pulmonary effects of short-term nose-only cigarette smoke exposure in mice. Experimental Biology and Medicine (Maywood, NJ). 2012;**237**(12):1449-1456

[87] Rinaldi M, et al. Long-term nose-only cigarette smoke exposure induces emphysema and mild skeletal muscle dysfunction in mice. Disease Models & Mechanisms. 2012;**5**(3):333-341

[88] Dvorkin-Gheva A, et al. Total particulate matter concentration skews cigarette smoke's gene expression profile. ERJ Open Research. eCollection 2016 Oct;**2**(4): pii: 00029-2016

[89] Gaschler GJ, et al. Cigarette smoke exposure attenuates cytokine production by mouse alveolar macrophages. American Journal of Respiratory Cell and Molecular Biology. 2008;**38**(2):218-226

[90] Raza H, John A, Nemmar A. Short-term effects of nose-only cigarette smoke exposure on glutathione redox homeostasis, cytochrome P450 1A1/2 and respiratory enzyme activities in mice tissues. Cellular Physiology and Biochemistry. 2013;**31**(4-5):683-692

[91] Beckett EL, et al. A new short-term mouse model of chronic obstructive pulmonary disease identifies a role for mast cell tryptase in pathogenesis. Journal of Allergy and Clinical Immunology. 2013;**131**(3):752-762

[92] Brown BG, et al. The effect of a 2-h exposure to cigarette smoke on the metabolic activation of the tobacco-specific nitrosamine 4-(methylnitrosamino)-1-(3-pyridyl)-1-butanone in A/J mice. Chemico-Biological Interactions. 2001;**138**(2):125-135

[93] Hamm JT, et al. Histological alterations in male A/J mice following nose-only exposure to tobacco smoke. Inhalation Toxicology. 2007;**19**(5):405-418

[94] Nemmar A, et al. Short-term systemic effects of nose-only cigarette smoke exposure in mice: Role of oxidative stress. Cellular Physiology and Biochemistry. 2013;**31**(1):15-24

[95] Foronjy RF, et al. Structural emphysema does not correlate with lung compliance: Lessons from the mouse smoking model. Experimental Lung Research. 2005;**31**(6):547-562

[96] Shalaby KH, et al. Combined forced oscillation and forced expiration measurements in mice for the assessment of airway hyperresponsiveness. Respiratory Research. 2010;**11**:82

[97] Golovatch P, et al. Role for cathepsin K in emphysema in smoke-exposed guinea pigs. Experimental Lung Research. 2009;**35**(8):631-645

[98] Geraghty P, Wallace A, D'Armiento JM. Induction of the unfolded protein response by cigarette smoke is primarily an activating transcription factor 4-C/EBP homologous protein mediated process. International Journal of Chronic Obstructive Pulmonary Disease. 2011;**6**:309-319

[99] Dominguez-Fandos D, et al. Sildenafil in a cigarette smoke-induced model of COPD in the guinea-pig. The European Respiratory Journal. 2015;**46**(2):346-354

[100] Kratzer A, et al. Role of IL-18 in second-hand smoke-induced emphysema. American Journal of Respiratory Cell and Molecular Biology. 2013;**48**(6):725-732

[101] Xiao R, Goldklang MP, D'Armiento JM. Parenchymal airspace profiling: Sensitive quantification and characterization of lung structure evaluating parenchymal destruction. American Journal of Respiratory Cell and Molecular Biology. 2016;**55**(5):708-715

[102] Goldklang MP, et al. Single-photon emission computed tomography/computed tomography imaging in a rabbit model of emphysema reveals ongoing apoptosis in vivo. American Journal of Respiratory Cell and Molecular Biology. 2016;**55**(6):848-857

[103] Geraghty P, Dabo AJ, D'Armiento J, TLR4 protein contributes to cigarette smoke-induced matrix metalloproteinase-1 (MMP-1) expression in chronic obstructive pulmonary disease. Journal of Biological Chemistry. 2011;**286**(34):30211-30218

[104] Lemaitre V, Dabo AJ, D'Armiento J. Cigarette smoke components induce matrix metalloproteinase-1 in aortic endothelial cells through inhibition of mTOR signaling. Toxicological Sciences. 2011;**123**(2):542-549

[105] Sezer M, et al. Effects of caffeic acid phenethyl ester on the histopathological changes in the lungs of cigarette smoke-exposed rabbits. Basic and Clinical Pharmacology and Toxicology. 2007;**101**(3):187-191

[106] Imai K, et al. Human collagenase (matrix metalloproteinase-1) expression in the lungs of patients with emphysema. American Journal of Respiratory and Critical Care Medicine. 2001;**163**(3 Pt 1):786-791

[107] Zabetian M, Tahmoorespur M, Hosseini K. The applications of transgenic rabbits in agriculture and biomedicine. Journal of Animal and Veterinary Advances. 2011;**10**(6): 780-790

[108] Kamaruzaman NA, et al. The rabbit as a model for studying lung disease and stem cell therapy. BioMed Research International. 2013;**2013**:691830

[109] Gosker HR, et al. Extrapulmonary manifestations of chronic obstructive pulmonary disease in a mouse model of chronic cigarette smoke exposure. American Journal of Respiratory Cell and Molecular Biology. 2009;**40**(6):710-716

[110] Tang K, Wagner PD, Breen EC. TNF-alpha-mediated reduction in PGC-1alpha may impair skeletal muscle function after cigarette smoke exposure. Journal of Cellular Physiology. 2010;**222**(2):320-327

[111] Foronjy R, et al. TLR9 expression is required for the development of cigarette smoke-induced emphysema in mice. American Journal of Physiology - Lung Cellular and Molecular Physiology. 2016;**311**(1):L154-L166. DOI: 10.1152/ajplung.00073.2016

[112] Foronjy RF, et al. Respiratory syncytial virus infections enhance cigarette smoke induced COPD in mice. PLoS One. 2014;**9**(2):e90567

[113] Phillips B, et al. A 7-month cigarette smoke inhalation study in C57BL/6 mice demonstrates reduced lung inflammation and emphysema following smoking cessation or aerosol exposure from a prototypic modified risk tobacco product. Food and Chemical Toxicology. 2015;**80**:328-345

[114] Botelho FM, et al. IL-1alpha/IL-1R1 expression in chronic obstructive pulmonary disease and mechanistic relevance to smoke-induced neutrophilia in mice. PLoS One. 2011;**6**(12):e28457

[115] Cardoso JF, et al. Effects of cigarette smoke in mice wound healing is strain dependent. Toxicologic Pathology. 2007;**35**(7):890-896

[116] Braber S, et al. Inflammatory changes in the airways of mice caused by cigarette smoke exposure are only partially reversed after smoking cessation. Respiratory Research. 2010;**11**:99

[117] Geraghty P, Hardigan A, Foronjy RF. Cigarette smoke activates the proto-oncogene c-src to promote airway inflammation and lung tissue destruction. American Journal of Respiratory Cell and Molecular Biology. 2014;**50**(3):559-570

[118] Geraghty P, et al. HIV infection model of chronic obstructive pulmonary disease in mice. American Journal of Physiology - Lung Cellular and Molecular Physiology. 2017;**312**(4):L500-L509. DOI: 10.1152/ajplung.00431.2016

[119] Foronjy RF, et al. Protein tyrosine phosphatase 1B negatively regulates S100A9-mediated lung damage during respiratory syncytial virus exacerbations. Mucosal Immunology. 2016;**9**(5):1317-1329

[120] Su BH, et al. Prothymosin alpha overexpression contributes to the development of pulmonary emphysema. Nature Communications. 2013;**4**:1906

[121] Barreiro E, et al. Cigarette smoke-induced oxidative stress in skeletal muscles of mice. Respiratory Physiology & Neurobiology. 2012;**182**(1):9-17

[122] Pittilo RM, et al. Effects of cigarette smoking on the ultrastructure of rat thoracic aorta and its ability to produce prostacyclin. Thrombosis and Haemostasis. 1982;**48**(2):173-176

[123] Lee JH, et al. Simvastatin inhibits cigarette smoking-induced emphysema and pulmonary hypertension in rat lungs. American Journal of Respiratory and Critical Care Medicine. 2005;**172**(8):987-993

[124] Alving K, Fornhem C, Lundberg JM. Pulmonary effects of endogenous and exogenous nitric oxide in the pig: Relation to cigarette smoke inhalation. British Journal of Pharmacology. 1993;**110**(2):739-746

[125] Hernandez JA, et al. Pulmonary parenchymal defects in dogs following prolonged cigarette smoke exposure. The American Review of Respiratory Disease. 1966;**93**(1):78-83

[126] Auerbach O, et al. Emphysema produced in dogs by cigarette smoking. JAMA. 1967;**199**(4):241-246

[127] Cahan WG, Kirman D. An effective system and procedure for cigarette smoking by dogs. Journal of Surgical Research. 1968;**8**(12):567-575

[128] Schroeder T, et al. PET imaging of regional 18F-FDG uptake and lung function after cigarette smoke inhalation. Journal of Nuclear Medicine. 2007;**48**(3):413-419

[129] Morris DG, et al. Loss of integrin alpha(v)beta6-mediated TGF-beta activation causes Mmp12-dependent emphysema. Nature. 2003;**422**(6928):169-173

[130] Suga T, et al. Disruption of the klotho gene causes pulmonary emphysema in mice. Defect in maintenance of pulmonary integrity during postnatal life. American Journal of Respiratory Cell and Molecular Biology. 2000;**22**(1):26-33

[131] D'Armiento J, et al. Collagenase expression in the lungs of transgenic mice causes pulmonary emphysema. Cell. 1992;**71**(6):955-961

[132] Rangasamy T, et al. Genetic ablation of Nrf2 enhances susceptibility to cigarette smoke-induced emphysema in mice. The Journal of Clinical Investigation. 2004;**114**(9):1248-1259

[133] Geraghty P, et al. The glutathione peroxidase 1-protein tyrosine phosphatase 1B-protein phosphatase 2A axis. A key determinant of airway inflammation and alveolar destruction. American Journal of Respiratory Cell and Molecular Biology. 2013;**49**(5):721-730

[134] Duong C, et al. Glutathione peroxidase-1 protects against cigarette smoke-induced lung inflammation in mice. American Journal of Physiology - Lung Cellular and Molecular Physiology. 2010;**299**(3):L425-L433

[135] Chrusciel S, et al. Lack of transcription factor p53 exacerbates elastase-induced emphysema in mice. American Journal of Respiratory Cell and Molecular Biology. 2016;**54**(2):188-199

[136] Hautamaki RD, et al. Requirement for macrophage elastase for cigarette smoke-induced emphysema in mice. Science. 1997;**277**(5334):2002-2004

[137] Volonte D, et al. Caveolin-1 expression is required for the development of pulmonary emphysema through activation of the ATM-p53-p21 pathway. Journal of Biological Chemistry. 2009;**284**(9):5462-5466

[138] Seimetz M, et al. Inducible NOS inhibition reverses tobacco-smoke-induced emphysema and pulmonary hypertension in mice. Cell. 2011;**147**(2):293-305

[139] Churg A, et al. Tumor necrosis factor-alpha drives 70% of cigarette smoke-induced emphysema in the mouse. American Journal of Respiratory and Critical Care Medicine. 2004;**170**(5):492-498

[140] van der Deen M, et al. Reduced inflammatory response in cigarette smoke exposed Mrp1/Mdr1a/1b deficient mice. Respiratory Research. 2007;**8**:49

[141] Morrow JD, et al. Functional interactors of three genome-wide association study genes are differentially expressed in severe chronic obstructive pulmonary disease lung tissue. Scientific Reports. 2017;**7**:44232

[142] Hobbs BD, et al. Genetic loci associated with chronic obstructive pulmonary disease overlap with loci for lung function and pulmonary fibrosis. Nature Genetics. 2017;**49**(3):426-432

[143] Maeno T, et al. CD8+ T Cells are required for inflammation and destruction in cigarette smoke-induced emphysema in mice. The Journal of Immunology. 2007;**178**(12):8090-8096

[144] Foronjy RF, et al. Superoxide dismutase expression attenuates cigarette smoke- or elastase-generated emphysema in mice. American Journal of Respiratory and Critical Care Medicine. 2006;**173**(6):623-631

[145] Kang MJ, et al. IL-18 is induced and IL-18 receptor alpha plays a critical role in the pathogenesis of cigarette smoke-induced pulmonary emphysema and inflammation. The Journal of Immunology. 2007;**178**(3):1948-1959

[146] Miller M, et al. Adiponectin-deficient mice are protected against tobacco-induced inflammation and increased emphysema. American Journal of Physiology - Lung Cellular and Molecular Physiology. 2010;**299**(6):L834-L842

[147] Yao H, et al. Extracellular superoxide dismutase protects against pulmonary emphysema by attenuating oxidative fragmentation of ECM. Proceedings of the National Academy of Sciences of the United States of America. 2010;**107**(35):15571-15576

[148] Shan M, et al. Cigarette smoke induction of osteopontin (SPP1) mediates T(H)17 inflammation in human and experimental emphysema. Science Translational Medicine. 2012;**4**(117):117ra9

[149] Bozinovski S, et al. Innate cellular sources of interleukin-17A regulate macrophage accumulation in cigarette- smoke-induced lung inflammation in mice. Clinical Science (London). 2015;**129**(9):785-796

[150] Shore S, et al. Increased airway responsiveness to inhaled methacholine in a rat model of chronic bronchitis. American Journal of Respiratory and Critical Care Medicine. 1995;**151**(6):1931-1938

[151] Kodavanti UP, et al. The spontaneously hypertensive rat: An experimental model of sulfur dioxide-induced airways disease. Toxicological Sciences. 2006;**94**(1):193-205

[152] Miller ML, et al. Effect of exposure to 500 ppm sulfur dioxide on the lungs of the ferret. Respiration. 1985;**48**(4):346-354

[153] Long NC, et al. Airway hyperresponsiveness in a rat model of chronic bronchitis: Role of C fibers. American Journal of Respiratory and Critical Care Medicine. 1997;**155**(4): 1222-1229

[154] Wegmann M, et al. NO2-induced airway inflammation is associated with progressive airflow limitation and development of emphysema-like lesions in C57bl/6 mice. Experimental and Toxicological Pathology. 2005;**56**(6):341-350

[155] Rombout PJ, et al. Influence of exposure regimen on nitrogen dioxide-induced morphological changes in the rat lung. Environmental Research. 1986;**41**(2):466-480

[156] Parkinson DR, Stephens RJ. Morphological surface changes in the terminal bronchiolar region of NO2-exposed rat lung. Environmental Research. 1973;**6**(1):37-51

[157] Mudway IS, Kelly FJ. Ozone and the lung: A sensitive issue. Molecular Aspects of Medicine. 2000;**21**(1-2):1-48

[158] Cai C, et al. Prior SO_2 exposure promotes airway inflammation and subepithelial fibrosis following repeated ovalbumin challenge. Clinical and Experimental Allergy. 2008;**38**(10):1680-1687

[159] Peiser C, et al. Dopamine D2 receptor mRNA expression is increased in the jugular-nodose ganglia of rats with nitrogen dioxide-induced chronic bronchitis. Neuroscience Letters. 2009;**465**(2):143-146

[160] Foster JR, et al. A comparative study of the pulmonary effects of NO2 in the rat and hamster. British Journal of Experimental Pathology. 1985;**66**(2):193-204

[161] Rasmussen RE, et al. Effects of nitrogen dioxide on respiratory tract clearance in the ferret. Journal of Toxicology and Environment Health. 1994;**41**(1):109-120

[162] Ito M, et al. Effect of clenbuterol on sulfur dioxide-induced acute bronchitis in guinea pigs. Research Communications in Molecular Pathology and Pharmacology. 1995;**87**(2): 199-209

[163] Papi A, et al. Bronchopulmonary inflammation and airway smooth muscle hyperresponsiveness induced by nitrogen dioxide in guinea pigs. European Journal of Pharmacology. 1999;**374**(2):241-247

[164] Miyata T, et al. Effect of N-acetylneuraminic acid on respiratory tract secretion and inflammation in the bronchitic rabbit. Archives Internationales de Pharmacodynamie et de Thérapie. 1990;**304**:277-289

[165] Haydon GB, et al. Nitrogen dioxide-induced emphysema in rabbits. The American Review of Respiratory Disease. 1967;**95**(5):797-805

[166] Man SF, et al. Effects of SO_2 exposure on canine pulmonary epithelial functions. Experimental Lung Research. 1989;**15**(2):181-198

[167] Hine CH, et al. Pulmonary changes in animals exposed to nitrogen dioxide. Proceedings of the Western Pharmacology Society. 1964;**7**:19-22

[168] Zhang Y, et al. Intraperitoneal injection of cigarette smoke extract induced emphysema, and injury of cardiac and skeletal muscles in BALB/C mice. Experimental Lung Research. 2013;**39**(1):18-31

[169] Pillai SG, et al. Loci identified by genome-wide association studies influence different disease-related phenotypes in chronic obstructive pulmonary disease. American Journal of Respiratory and Critical Care Medicine. 2010;**182**(12):1498-1505

[170] Zia S, et al. Nicotine enhances expression of the alpha 3, alpha 4, alpha 5, and alpha 7 nicotinic receptors modulating calcium metabolism and regulating adhesion and motility of respiratory epithelial cells. Research Communications in Molecular Pathology and Pharmacology. 1997;**97**(3):243-262

[171] Maouche K, et al. {alpha}7 nicotinic acetylcholine receptor regulates airway epithelium differentiation by controlling basal cell proliferation. The American Journal of Pathology. 2009;**175**(5):1868-1882

[172] Diamond L, et al. Augmentation of elastase-induced emphysema by cigarette smoke. Effects of reduced nicotine content. The American Review of Respiratory Disease. 1988;**138**(5):1201-1206

[173] Xu Y, Zhang Y, Cardell LO. Nicotine exaggerates LPS-induced airway hyperreactivity via JNK-mediated up-regulation of toll-like receptor 4. American Journal of Respiratory Cell and Molecular Biology. 2014;**51**(3):370-379

[174] Paleari L, et al. Role of alpha7-nicotinic acetylcholine receptor in human non-small cell lung cancer proliferation. Cell Proliferation. 2008;**41**(6):936-959

[175] Services, U.S.D.o.H.a.H.. E-Cigarette Use Among Youth and Young Adults: A Report of the Surgeon General. Murthy VH, et al, 2016. https://e-cigarettes.surgeongeneral.gov/documents/2016_sgr_full_report_non-508.pdf

[176] Lerner CA, et al. Vapors produced by electronic cigarettes and e-juices with flavorings induce toxicity, oxidative stress, and inflammatory response in lung epithelial cells and in mouse lung. PLoS One. 2015;**10**(2):e0116732

[177] Sussan TE, et al. Exposure to electronic cigarettes impairs pulmonary anti-bacterial and anti-viral defenses in a mouse model. PLoS One. 2015;**10**(2):e0116861

[178] Garcia-Arcos I, et al. Chronic electronic cigarette exposure in mice induces features of COPD in a nicotine-dependent manner. Thorax. 2016;**71**(12):1119-1129

[179] Yoshizaki K, et al. Chronic exposure of diesel exhaust particles induces alveolar enlargement in mice. Respiratory Research. 2015;**16**:18

[180] Mehra D, et al. A comparison of the inflammatory and proteolytic effects of dung biomass and cigarette smoke exposure in the lung. PLoS One. 2012;**7**(12):e52889

[181] Shapiro D, et al. Activation of transient receptor potential ankyrin-1 (TRPA1) in lung cells by wood smoke particulate material. Chemical Research in Toxicology. 2013;**26**(5):750-758

[182] Organization, W.H. Household Air Pollution and Health; WHO Organization; 2016. http://www.who.int/mediacentre/factsheets/fs292/en/

[183] Donaldson GC, et al. Factors associated with change in exacerbation frequency in COPD. Respiratory Research. 2013;**14**:79

[184] Seemungal TA, et al. Detection of rhinovirus in induced sputum at exacerbation of chronic obstructive pulmonary disease. The European Respiratory Journal. 2000;**16**(4):677-683

[185] Stockley RA, et al. Relationship of sputum color to nature and outpatient management of acute exacerbations of COPD. Chest. 2000;**117**(6):1638-1645

[186] Sakhatskyy P, et al. Double-hit mouse model of cigarette smoke priming for acute lung injury. American Journal of Physiology - Lung Cellular and Molecular Physiology. 2017;**312**(1):L56-L67

[187] Mizutani N, et al. Pulmonary emphysema induced by cigarette smoke solution and lipopolysaccharide in guinea pigs. Biological and Pharmaceutical Bulletin. 2009;**32**(9): 1559-1564

[188] Huvenne W, et al. Exacerbation of cigarette smoke-induced pulmonary inflammation by *Staphylococcus aureus* enterotoxin B in mice. Respiratory Research. 2011;**12**:69

[189] Kang MJ, et al. Cigarette smoke selectively enhances viral PAMP- and virus-induced pulmonary innate immune and remodeling responses in mice. The Journal of Clinical Investigation. 2008;**118**(8):2771-2784

[190] Kimura G, et al. Toll-like receptor 3 stimulation causes corticosteroid-refractory airway neutrophilia and hyperresponsiveness in mice. Chest. 2013;**144**(1):99-105

[191] Kearley J, et al. Cigarette smoke silences innate lymphoid cell function and facilitates an exacerbated type I interleukin-33-dependent response to infection. Immunity. 2015;**42**(3):566-579

[192] Sajjan U, et al. Elastase- and LPS-exposed mice display altered responses to rhinovirus infection. American Journal of Physiology - Lung Cellular and Molecular Physiology. 2009;**297**(5):L931-L944

[193] Takahashi S, et al. Pneumococcal infection aggravates elastase-induced emphysema via matrix metalloproteinase 12 overexpression. Journal of Infectious Diseases. 2016;**213**(6):1018-1030

[194] Potash MJ, et al. A mouse model for study of systemic HIV-1 infection, antiviral immune responses, and neuroinvasiveness. Proceedings of the National Academy of Sciences of the United States of America. 2005;**102**(10):3760-3765

[195] Diaz PT, et al. Increased susceptibility to pulmonary emphysema among HIV-seropositive smokers. Annals of Internal Medicine. 2000;**132**(5):369-372

[196] Crothers K, et al. Increased COPD among HIV-positive compared to HIV-negative veterans. Chest. 2006;**130**(5):1326-1333

[197] Gingo MR, Morris A, Crothers K. Human immunodeficiency virus-associated obstructive lung diseases. Clinics in Chest Medicine. 2013;**34**(2):273-282

[198] Drummond MB, Kirk GD. HIV-associated obstructive lung diseases: Insights and implications for the clinician. The Lancet Respiratory Medicine. 2014;**2**(7):583-592

[199] Gaschler GJ, et al. Bacteria challenge in smoke-exposed mice exacerbates inflammation and skews the inflammatory profile. American Journal of Respiratory and Critical Care Medicine. 2009;**179**(8):666-675

[200] Gaschler GJ, et al. Mechanisms of clearance of nontypeable *Haemophilus influenzae* from cigarette smoke-exposed mouse lungs. The European Respiratory Journal. 2010;**36**(5):1131-1142

[201] Sun L, et al. The effect and mechanism of action of carbocysteine on airway bacterial load in rats chronically exposed to cigarette smoke. Respirology. 2010;**15**(7):1064-1071

[202] Barnes PJ, Celli BR. Systemic manifestations and comorbidities of COPD. The European Respiratory Journal. 2009;**33**(5):1165-1185

[203] Sin DD, Man SF. Chronic obstructive pulmonary disease as a risk factor for cardiovascular morbidity and mortality. Proceedings of the American Thoracic Society. 2005;**2**(1):8-11

[204] Chatila WM, et al. Comorbidities in chronic obstructive pulmonary disease. Proceedings of the American Thoracic Society. 2008;**5**(4):549-555

[205] Chen H, et al. Cigarette smoke exposure reprograms the hypothalamic neuropeptide Y axis to promote weight loss. American Journal of Respiratory and Critical Care Medicine. 2006;**173**(11):1248-1254

[206] Hu N, et al. Cardiac-specific overexpression of metallothionein rescues against cigarette smoking exposure-induced myocardial contractile and mitochondrial damage. PLoS One. 2013;**8**(2):e57151

[207] Sussan TE, et al. Targeting Nrf2 with the triterpenoid CDDO-imidazolide attenuates cigarette smoke-induced emphysema and cardiac dysfunction in mice. Proceedings of the National Academy of Sciences of the United States of America. 2009;**106**(1):250-255

[208] Talukder MA, et al. Chronic cigarette smoking causes hypertension, increased oxidative stress, impaired NO bioavailability, endothelial dysfunction, and cardiac remodeling in mice. American Journal of Physiology - Heart and Circulatory Physiology. 2011;**300**(1):H388-H396

[209] Antunes MA, et al. Effects of different mesenchymal stromal cell sources and delivery routes in experimental emphysema. Respiratory Research. 2014;**15**:118

[210] Hoffmann D, Hecht SS, Wynder EL. Tumor promoters and cocarcinogens in tobacco carcinogenesis. Environmental Health Perspectives. 1983;**50**:247-257

[211] Cosio M, et al. The relations between structural changes in small airways and pulmonary-function tests. The New England Journal of Medicine. 1978;**298**(23):1277-1281

[212] Jobse BN, et al. Impact of inflammation, emphysema, and smoking cessation on V/Q in mouse models of lung obstruction. Respiratory Research. 2014;**15**:42

Chapter 2

Genetics Association and Epigenetic Changes in COPD

Rajneesh Malhotra and Outi Vaarala

Additional information is available at the end of the chapter

http://dx.doi.org/10.5772/intechopen.72439

Abstract

Genome-wide association studies (GWASs) have successfully identified susceptibility loci associated with COPD. The genes mapped on these loci, eg The FAM13A gene (family with sequence similarity 13, member A), provide a new approach to understand the COPD pathology. Furthermore, heavy smoking is reported to correlate with altered methylation and epigenetic changes of multiple genes in small airway cells. These changes have been shown to be associated with the severity of COPD. It is likely that smoking-induced changes in epigenetic control of gene expression result in genetically vulnerable individual's results in reduced tissue repair, tissue damage and persistent inflammation associated with COPD pathophysiology.

Keywords: microRNA, acetylation, GWAS, bromodomain

1. Introduction

Chronic obstructive pulmonary disease (COPD) is characterized by sustained inflammation of the airways, leading to destruction of lung tissue and declining pulmonary function. In COPD the repetitive challenges to the lung, due to external environmental insults, cause chronic inflammation of the bronchi and small airways leading to destruction of lung tissue (emphysema), as well as scarring (remodeling and fibrosis). The inflammatory process in COPD is characterized by predominant increase in neutrophils and macrophages in the lung and an upregulation of proinflammatory cytokines, including TNF-a, IL-1, IL-6, IL-8, IL-18, IL-17 and IL-32 [1]. Such failure to resolve inflammation and initiate proper repair causes permanent structural damage and perturbations in tissue cellular composition resulting in chronic disease [2, 3]. Smoking is the risk factor for COPD but only about 20% of smokers develop COPD [3], indicating that while smoking is an important cause or initiating factor, it is not the only driver of disease progression in COPD patients. In this chapter, we explore the principles for the interplay between genetics and environmental factors induced epigenetic changes in the etiology and pathology of COPD pathophysiology.

2. Genetics

SERPINA1 mutation was the first fully defined genetic risk associated with chronic obstructive pulmonary diseases. SERPINA1 is the gene encoding alpha-1 antitrypsin (AAT) and systemic deficiency in AAT (AATD) due to genetic mutations can result in liver failure and chronic lung disease such as emphysema (4). AAT is the most abundant circulating serine protease inhibitor (serpin) and an acute phase reactant. The emphysema observed in patients with AATD, consisting of progressive destruction of the alveoli and small airway structure, formed the basis of the protease/anti-protease imbalance theory of chronic obstructive pulmonary disease (COPD).

Alpha-1 antitrypsin deficiency (AATD) is an inherited disorder and its role in lung emphysema was established by studying the phenotype of the patients [4]. The single candidate gene provides association for a gene in host physiology, whereas Genome-wide association studies (GWAS) identifies genome-wide set of genetic variants to a complex disease. Recently, significant progress is been made to understand the function of the genes associated with the Single nucleotide polymorphisms (SNP's) in the susceptible loci for COPD. One such COPD disease susceptibility locus is in the nicotinic acetylcholine receptor (nAChR) gene cluster CHRNA5-A3-B4 on the long arm of chromosome 15 (15q24–25.1), indicating a link to COPD is through effects on smoking behavior. nAChRs provide binding sites for nicotine and regulates nicotine mediated effects in the brain. For instance, it is been documents that smokers carrying the rs16969968 risk allele in CHRNA5 are likely to smoke more heavily than their counterparts without the risk allele. Due to increased habit of smoking these individuals run an increased risk of impaired epithelial barrier function and development of COPD due to increased smoke exposure. The CHRNA3/CHRNA5 locus has also been identified in genome-wide association studies in lung cancer and other diseases significantly influenced by cigarette smoking behavior and exposure [5, 6, 7].

Another susceptibility locus on chromosome 15 (15q25.1) is in the IREB2 gene, encoding the protein IRP2 (iron-responsive element-binding proteins), which is involved in maintaining human cellular iron metabolism. Interestingly, accumulation of iron in the lungs of healthy smokers and smokers with COPD has been reported [8], and the same has been observed in people exposed to particulate air pollutions [9]. This may be important as tight regulation of iron homeostasis is crucial not only to maintain normal cellular function, but also to prevent iron-mediated oxidative stress and damage [10]. Oxidative stress is suggested to be a key driver of pathogenesis in COPD [10], and reactive oxygen species (ROS) generated in the presence of an excess of free iron via the Fenton reaction [10] may be an important cause of cellular and tissue damage in the COPD lung.

GWAS has also identified COPD susceptibility loci on chromosome 4 in 4q22 (FAM13) and 4q31 (HHIP). FAM13A (also known as FAM13A1) is suggested to have a putative role in signal transduction in response to hypoxia. The most statistically significant SNPs are in an intronic region downstream of a Rho GTPase–activating protein (RhoGAP) domain [11], COPD risk alleles at the FAM13A locus is reported to be associated with increased expression of FAM13A in human lungs. In a recent publication it was reported that in murine and human lungs, FAM13A is expressed in airway and alveolar type II epithelial cells and macrophages [12]. Furthermore, the authors reported that Fam13a null mice (Fam13a2/2) were resistant to chronic cigarette smoke–induced emphysema compared with Fam13a expressing mice. It was shown that FAM13A modulates catenin pathway by interacting with protein phosphatase 2A and recruits protein phosphatase 2A to regulate glycogen synthase kinase 3β activity resulting in β-catenin degradation. These results indicate that FAM13A could increase the susceptibility of mice to emphysema development by inhibiting β-catenin signaling. β-catenin signaling activates the expression of Wnt target genes that promote cell proliferation and limit cell differentiation [11]. In the absence of FAM13A, β-catenin pathway is restored leading to a more effective lung repair program in lung alveolar epithelial cells after CS exposure. This hypothesis was further supported by expression data, indicating increased FAM13A protein levels and decreased β-catenin protein levels in human COPD lung tissues compared with ex-smokers without COPD [11, 12].

These observations provide evidence for potential role for these pathways in COPD patients with emphysema and potential for utilizing SNP's associated with FAM13A for patient stratification for drugs modulating catenin pathway. Increased levels of FAM13A blocks the pathways associated with lung regeneration, therefore inhibition or deletion of FAM13A in COPD patients with risk allele at the FAM13A locus could be a potential way to induce epithelium regeneration in emphysematic patients.

In two independent genome-wide association studies, Hedgehog interacting protein (HHIP) was identified as a COPD susceptibility gene in subjects from the Framingham Heart Study and a homogenous case control cohort from Norway, respectively [13, 14]. The SNPs map to an intergenic region upstream of the HHIP gene and regulates HHIP gene expression in carriers. HHIP is expressed in epithelial cells and considered to modulate epithelial barrier structure as reported by Zhou et al. [15]. Zhou and workers [15] reported that modulation of HHIP expression results in differential expression of 296 epithelial genes, most of which associated with ECM matrix interactions, junctional complexes or cell growth. Analysis of epithelial cells derived from human lung tissue showed significantly decreased expression of these genes in cells from COPD patients as compared to cells from healthy controls. These observations indicate loss of HHIP function in human bronchial epithelial cells may contribute to susceptibility to smoke-induced COPD by regulating genes important for epithelial barrier integrity and function [15].

In a recent meta-analysis study, Busch and coworkers [16] genotyped 3346 single nucleotide polymorphisms (SNP) in 2588 cases (1803 severe COPD) and 1782 controls from four cohorts. They analyzed association testing with COPD, combining their results with existing genotyping data from 6633 cases (3497 severe COPD) and 5704 controls. In this analysis, authors confirmed significance of previously documented SNPs in the Transforming growth factor beta 2 (TGFB2), FAM13A, HHIP, Matrix metalloproteinases 3 (MMP3)/Matrix metalloproteinases 12 (MMP12), and CHRNA3/CHRNA5/IREB2 regions with COPD pathophysiology. Authors identified two SNPs at loci not previously identified. These two loci showed significant associations between SNPs near PPIC and PPP4R4/SERPINA1 and severe COPD.

The GWAS analysis has indicated genes associated in COPD pathophysiology. In the future further investigation of specific pathophysiology regulated by genes associated with SNP's may allow patient stratification based on genetic linkage and development of drugs to modulate disease phenotype.

3. Epigenetics of COPD

Epigenetics is defined as study of heritable changes in gene expression resulting in change in cellular phenotype caused by mechanisms that do not alter the Deoxyribonucleic acid (DNA) sequence. Epigenetic modifications control gene expression by changes to the structure and function of chromatin. Environmental challenges such as cigarette smoke, can lead to permanent changes in epigenetic patterns (epimutations) resulting in development of chronic disease. Examples of such epigenetic mechanisms include DNA methylation, histone modification and RNA interference [17].

DNA methylation is a process resulting in the covalent addition of a methyl group to cytosine residues part of cytosine-guanine (CpG) dinucleotides, and when a gene is methylated on CpG islands in promoter areas, transcriptional repression is generally the result, representing an important mechanism for gene silencing. In patients with COPD some loci are identified as hypermethylated and other hypomethylation [18–20]. The loci identified to be hypermethylated are reported to be Genes components of the PI3K/Akt and anti-oxidant NFE2-related factor-2 (Nrf2) pathways [20]. The CpG hypermethylation observed in the PTEN and NFE2L2 (Nrf2) genes correlates with reduced expression of their respective gene products. The Nrf2 pathway is anti-inflammatory and protects against oxidative stress, whereas PTEN is a negative regulator of PI3K/AKT signaling, contributes to inflammation, remodeling, and proteolysis in COPD. Thus, CpG hypermethylation appears to antagonize protective pathways regulating pathophysiology of COPD. On the other hand, hypomethylation of the HDAC6 promoter has been linked to elevated expression of HDAC6 in COPD [21]. HDAC6 is thought to contribute to cigarette smoke-mediated epithelial dysfunction in COPD by promoting autophagy [21].

Posttranscriptional modifications to histone ends in the histone H3 and H4 residues define the accessibility of the chromatin to the different coactivators or corepressors. Histone acetylation is regulated by the levels and activities of histone acetyl transferases (HAT) and histone deacetylases (HDAC). Increase in HAT activity results in increased acetylation of lysine residues in histones and gene transcription, whereas as increase in HDAC activity negatively regulates gene transcription. Simplistically, chromatin is transcriptionally active when lysines on histones H3 and H4 are acetylated.

It has been proposed that the inhibition of HDAC2 activity also contributes to the glucocorticoid resistance seen in COPD inflammation [22–24]. In lung biopsies obtained from COPD patients reduced HDAC2 activity and increased acetylation of histones have been reported [25]. The reduced HDAC2 expression and activity is shown to be associated with increased acetylation of histones H2A, H2B, H3, and H4 in the lungs and alveolar macrophages of COPD patients [26]. Yang et al. [27] reported that chronic cigarette smoke (CS) results epigenetic modifications of histone causing abnormal and sustained lung inflammatory response that occurs in smokers and in patients with COPD. They reported increased levels of KC, MCP-1, IL-6, and GM-CSF in mouse lung homogenate at both 3 days and 8 weeks of CS exposure in mice. Furthermore, they demonstrated using Chromatin immunoprecipitation (ChIP)-sequencing in CS exposed mouse lung that pro-inflammatory gene expression was due to the increased phosphorylation/acetylation of specific histone H3 (lys9/ser10) and histone H4 (lys12) in the promoter region of pro-inflammatory gene. Chen et al. [28] reported that cigarette smoke decreased the levels of HDAC1 expression and increased H3K9 acetylation. These modifications were associated with altered expression of pro-inflammatory mediators in CS-induced rat lungs and in macrophages.

These reported altered activity of HDAC's with increased histone acetylation in preclinical models and alveolar macrophages from COPD patients points to a potential role for epigenetic pathways in chronic lung inflammation in COPD patients.

Taken together these studies indicate that an imbalance between histone acetylases and deacetylases contributes to disease specific alterations in gene expression.

Sirtuin-1 (SIRT1) expression and deacetylase activity are reduced in peripheral lung tissues from patients with COPD [29, 30]. Reduced SIRT1 activity correlated with increased expression of MMP9 and H4 pan-acetylation [29]. Recently, Baker et al. [24] reported that oxidative stress (hydrogen peroxide) induces reduction of SIRT1/−6 in bronchial epithelial cells (BEAS2B). SIRT1 is reported to inhibits autophagy, cellular senescence, fibrosis, and inflammation by deacetylation of target proteins using NAD^+ as co-substrate. Similarly SIRT6 have also been shown to be associated with reduction–oxidation reaction (redox) state and inhibits cellular senescence and fibrosis [31]. Therefore, pathways associated with activation of SIRT1 and SIRT6 are an attractive approach for novel therapeutic targets for COPD. In the preclinical models efficacy of non-selective activators of SIRT1 using the pharmacological activator SRT1720 has been demonstrated Activation of SIRT1 via SRT2172 inhibits pulmonary neutrophil accumulation, and completely restored exercise tolerance and the fall in oxygen saturation and protects against cigarette smoke (CS) and elastase-induced emphysema in mice [32]. Furthermore, resveratrol, a substance shown to activate SIRT1 attenuates cigarette smoke extract (CSE)-mediated glutathione depletion through reversing CSE-mediated NRF2 carbonylation in lung epithelium cell line, A549 cells [31, 32]. Due to a recent study in human airway smooth muscle cells, resveratrol is suggested as an anti-inflammatory therapy alternative to corticosteroids in COPD, particularly in COPD exacerbations [33].

The family of acetylation binding module termed as bromodomain recognizes acetylation sites on chromatin and was identified in the early 1990s in the brahma gene from *Drosophila melanogaster* [34]. The human proteome encodes 61 bromodomains, which are present in 46 diverse nuclear and cytoplasmic proteins. The BET (bromodomain and extra-terminal) proteins (BRD2, BRD3, BRDT and BRD4) belong to this family of bromodomain containing proteins. BET proteins bind to acetylated lysines in the histones of nucleosomal chromatin and function either as co-activators or co-repressor of gene expression [34]. Due to the hyperacetylation patterns observed in COPD the modulation of BET (bromodomain and extra-terminal) proteins are new targets in modulating pathophysiology in patients. Nicodeme et al. [35] reported that a synthetic compound I-BET, a potent inhibitor of bromodomain-containing BET proteins to acetylated histones, dissociates the formation of the chromatin complexes essential for the LPS-induced expression of inflammatory cytokines in a temporal manner (early middle and late response). Recently, we proposed that inhibition of BET protein interactions with hyperacetylated sites in the chromatin will regulate excessive activation of pro-inflammatory genes and survival of inflammatory cells associated with inflammation in COPD. We demonstrated for the first time a known BET inhibitor, JQ1, showed a difference potency for inhibitions of IL6 in human peripheral blood mononuclear cells (PBMC) from normal or COPD in comparison to alveolar macrophages stimulated with LPS [31]. Furthermore, BET inhibitor JQ1 attenuated multiple genes, including pro-inflammatory cytokines and genes regulating innate and adaptive immune cells. We have used the set of genes modulated by JQ1 to generate a gene signature defining BET regulated genes [34]. Analysis of the expression of these gene signature genes,10 genes - CMPK2, EPSTI1, IFI44, IFI44L, IFIT1, IFIT3, MX1, OAS2, RSAD2 and XAF1, in the COPD samples compared to samples from normal controls, a subset of COPD patients with increased expression of these signature genes were identified. These results indicates that epigenetic modification associated gene expression could be utilized to do patient stratification and identify patients likely to show maximum response to given epigenetic modulator.

Nimmo and coworkers [36] have reported the co-localization of differentially methylated CpG regions and predisposing SNPs identified by GWAS in Crohn's disease. They observed methylations within 50 kilobases from several GWAS susceptibility loci, including IL-27, IL-19, TNF, MST1, and NOD2. A similar analysis in COPD is yet to be conducted. An analysis of epigenetic modification of genes identified by GWAS in COPD, including low probability associations, could highlight key pathways and points of regulation involved in the disease pathology, enabling target identification, patient stratification and prediction of treatment response.

4. MicroRNA-silencing RNA

A microRNA (miRNA) is a small non-coding RNA molecule (containing about 22 nucleotides) found in plants, animals and some viruses, that regulates the expression of complementary RNA thus functions in RNA silencing and post-transcriptional regulation of gene expression [37]. The expression of miRNAs are generally downregulated in smokers compared to non-smokers in airway epithelium [38], alveolar macrophages [39] and in lung tissue [40]. Dicer is an enzyme that cleaves pre-microRNA (pre-miRNA) into microRNA [41]. It is proposed that smoking downmodulated Dicer activity following sumoylation of Dicer resulting in down-modulation of miRNA in smokers [41]. Microarray-based studies have identified a large number of differentially expressed miRNAs in primary fibroblasts and lung tissue from patients with COPD [40–42]. Many of the miRNAs implicated in COPD have also been associated with various cancers, whereas miRNA that discriminated COPD from lung cancer have also been identified, including miRNAs 26a, 641, 383, 940, 662, 92a, 369-5p, and 636 [43] and miRNAs 20a, 24, 25, 152, 145, 199a [43]. Reduced expression of miR-199a-5p was reported in regulatory T cells from patients with COPD. miR-199a-5p targets genes includes members of the TGFβ superfamily [44] therefore plays a role in T-regulatory cells (Treg) cell function. Reduced miR-199a-5p expression in regulatory T cells in COPD may enhance regulatory T cell function resulting in abnormal bias towards Th1 immune responses [44]. Therefore, dysregulated miRNAs are potential treatment targets in COPD although additional studies are warranted to help determine whether observed differences in miRNAs are a cause or consequence of COPD.

http://dx.doi.org/10.5772/intechopen.72439

5. Conclusion

The chronic exposure to cigarette smoke or other air pollutants possibly induce epigenetic modifications, changes in lung cellular microenvironment and epithelial dysfunction. This may pathogens and to drive structural damage and changes in tissue cellular architecture typical of chronic inflammatory disease. Further research is required to map the specific epigenetic changes in lung tissue obtained from COPD patients, and combine this data with a detailed analysis of the disease pathophysiology to identify specific targets and patient stratification biomarker for modulating symptoms in COPD.

Author details

Rajneesh Malhotra* and Outi Vaarala

*Address all correspondence to: rajneesh.malhotra@astrazeneca.com

Immunity Department, RIA IMED Biotech Unit, AstraZeneca Gothenburg, Mölndal, Sweden

References

[1] Atamas SP, Chapoval SP, Keegan AD. Cytokines in chronic respiratory diseases. F1000 Biology Reports. 2013;**5**:3-10

[2] Barnes PJ. Chronic obstructive pulmonary disease. The New England Journal of Medicine. 2000;**343**:269-280

[3] Silverman EK. Progress in chronic obstructive pulmonary disease genetics. Proceedings of the American Thoracic Society. 2006;**3**:405-408

[4] Greene CM, Marciniak SJ, Teckman J, Ferrarotti I, Brantly ML, Lomas DA, Stoller JK, McElvaney NG. α1-antitrypsin deficiency. Nature Reviews Disease Primers. 2016 Jul 28;**2**: 16051. DOI: 10.1038/nrdp.2016.51

[5] El-Zein RA, Young RP, Hopkins RJ, Etzel CJ. Genetic predisposition to chronic obstructive pulmonary disease and/or lung cancer: Important considerations when evaluating risk. Cancer Prevention Research. 2012;**5**(4):522-527

[6] Bierut LJ, Stitzel JA, Wang JC, Hinrichs AL, Grucza RA, Xuei X, Saccone NL, Saccone SF, Bertelsen S, Fox L, Horton WJ, Breslau N, Budde J, Cloninger CR, Dick DM, Foroud T, Hatsukami D, Hesselbrock V, Johnson EO, Kramer J, Kuperman S, Madden PA, Mayo K, Nurnberger J Jr, Pomerleau O, Porjesz B, Reyes O, Schuckit M, Swan G, Tischfield JA, Edenberg HJ, Rice JP, Goate AM. Variants in nicotinic receptors and risk for nicotine dependence. American Journal of Psychiatry. 2008;**165**:1163-1171

[7] Ware JJ, van den Bree M, Munafò MR. From men to mice: CHRNA5/CHRNA3, smoking behavior and disease. Nicotine & Tobacco Research. 2012;**14**:1291-1299

[8] Ghio AJ, Hilborn ED, Stonehuerner JG, Dailey LA, Carter JD, Richards JH, Crissman KM, Foronjy RF, Uyeminami DL, Pinkerton KE. Particulate matter in cigarette smoke alters iron homeostasis to produce a biological effect. American Journal of Respiratory and Critical Care Medicine. 2008;**178**:1130-1138

[9] Ghio AJ, Cohen MD. Disruption of iron homeostasis as a mechanism of biologic effect by ambient air pollution particles. Inhalation Toxicology. 2005;**17**(13):709-716

[10] McGuinness AJ, Sapey E. Oxidative stress in COPD: Sources, markers, and potential mechanisms. Journal of Clinical Medicine. 2017 Feb 15;**6**(2). pii: E21). DOI: 10.3390/jcm6020021

[11] Cho MH, Boutaoui N, Klanderman BJ, Sylvia JS, Ziniti JP, Hersh CP, DeMeo DL, Hunninghake GM, Litonjua AA, Sparrow D, Lange C, Won S, Murphy JR, Beaty TH, Regan EA, Make BJ, Hokanson JE, Crapo JD, Kong X, Anderson WH, Tal-Singer R, Lomas DA, Bakke P, Gulsvik A, Pillai SG, Silverman EK. Variants in FAM13A are associated with chronic obstructive pulmonary disease. Nature Genetics. 2010;**42**:200-2002

[12] Jiang Z, Lao T, Qiu W, Polverino F, Gupta K, Guo F, Mancini JD, Naing ZZ, Cho MH, Castaldi PJ, Sun Y, Yu J, Laucho-Contreras ME, Kobzik L, Raby BA, Choi AM, Perrella MA, Owen CA, Silverman EK, Zhou X. A chronic obstructive pulmonary disease susceptibility gene, FAM13A, regulates protein stability of β-catenin. American Journal of Respiratory and Critical Care Medicine. 2016 Jul 15;**194**:185-197

[13] Wilk JB, Chen TH, Gottlieb DJ, et al. A genome-wide association study of pulmonary function measures in the Framingham heart study. PLoS Genetics. 2009;**5**(3):1170-1173

[14] Pillai SG, Ge D, Zhu G, et al. ICGN investigators. A genome-wide association study in chronic obstructive pulmonary disease (COPD): Identification of two major susceptibility loci. PLoS Genetics. 2009;**5**(3):1498-1505

[15] Zhou X, Qiu W, Sathirapongsasuti JF, Cho MH, Mancini JD, Lao T, Thibault DM, Litonjua AA, Bakke PS, Gulsvik A, Lomas DA, Beaty TH, Hersh CP, Anderson C, Geigenmuller U, Raby BA, Rennard SI, Perrella MA, Choi AM, Quackenbush J, Silverman EK. Gene expression analysis uncovers novel hedgehog interacting protein (HHIP) effects in human bronchial epithelial cells. Genomics. 2013;**101**(5):263-272

[16] Busch R, Hobbs BD, Zhou J, Castaldi PJ, McGeachie MJ, Hardin ME, Hawrylkiewicz I, Sliwinski P, Yim JJ, Kim WJ, Kim DK, Agusti A, Make BJ, Crapo JD, Calverley PM, Donner CF, Lomas DA, Wouters EF, Vestbo J, Tal-Singer R, Bakke P, Gulsvik A, Litonjua AA, Sparrow D, Paré PD, Levy RD, Rennard SI, Beaty TH, Hokanson J, Silverman EK, Cho MH. NETT genetics, ECLIPSE, ICGN, and COPDGene investigators. Genetic association and risk scores in a COPD meta-analysis of 16,707 subjects. American Journal of Respiratory Cell and Molecular Biology. 2017 Feb 7. DOI: 10.1165/rcmb.2016-0331OC

[17] Arrowsmith CH, Bountra C, Fish PV, Lee K, Schapira M. Epigenetic protein families: A new frontier for drug discovery. Nature Drug Discovery. 2012;**11**:384-400

[18] Liu F, Killian JK, Yang M, et al. Epigenomic alterations and gene expression profiles in respiratory epithelia exposed to cigarette smoke condensate. Oncogene. 2010;**29**(25): 3650-3664

[19] Qiu W, Baccarelli A, Carey VJ, et al. Variable DNA methylation is associated with chronic obstructive pulmonary disease and lung function. American Journal of Respiratory and Critical Care Medicine. 2012;**185**(4):373-381

[20] Vucic EA, Chari R, Thu KL, Wilson IM, Cotton AM, Kennett JY, Zhang M, Lonergan KM, Steiling K, Brown CJ, McWilliams A, Ohtani K, Lenburg ME, Sin DD, Spira A, Macaulay CE, Lam S, Lam WL. DNA methylation is globally disrupted and associated with expression changes in chronic obstructive pulmonary disease small airways. American Journal of Respiratory Cell and Molecular Biology. 2014 May;**50**(5):912-922

[21] Lam HC, Cloonan SM, Bhashyam AR, et al. Histone deacetylase 6-mediated selective autophagy regulates COPD associated cilia dysfunction. The Journal of Clinical Investigation. 2013;**123**(12):5212-5230

[22] Barnes PJ, Adcock IM, Ito K. Histone acetylation and deacetylation: Importance in inflammatory lung diseases. The European Respiratory Journal. 2005;**25**:552-563

[23] Barnes PJ. Reduced histone deacetylase in COPD: Clinical implications. Chest. 2006;**129**: 151-155

[24] Barnes PJ. Targeting the epigenome in the treatment of asthma and chronic obstructive pulmonary disease. Proceedings of the American Thoracic Society. 2009;**6**:693-696

[25] Ito K, Ito M, Elliott WM, Cosio B, Caramori G, Kon OM, Barczyk A, Hayashi S, Adcock IM, Hogg JC, Barnes PJ. Decreased histone deacetylase activity in chronic obstructive pulmonary disease. The New England Journal of Medicine. 2005;**352**:1967-1976

[26] Chen ZH, Kim HP, Sciurba FC, Lee SJ, Feghali-Bostwick C, Stolz DB, Dhir R, Landreneau RJ, Schuchert MJ, Yousem SA, Nakahira K, Pilewski JM, Lee JS, Zhang Y, Ryter SW, Choi AM. Egr-1 regulates autophagy in cigarette smoke-induced chronic obstructive pulmonary disease. PLoS One. 2009;**3**:e3316

[27] Yang S, Valvo S, Yao H, Kode A, Rajendrasozhan S, Edirisinghe I, et al. IKKα causes chromatin modification on pro-inflammatory genes by cigarette smoke in mouse lung. American Journal of Respiratory Cell and Molecular Biology. 2008;**38**:689-698

[28] Chen Z, Kim HP, Sciurba FC, Lee S, Feghali-Bostwick C, Stolz DB, et al. Egr-1 regulates autophagy in cigarette smoke-induced chronic obstructive pulmonary disease. PLoS One. 2008;**3**:e3316. DOI: 10.1371/journal.pone.0003316

[29] Nakamaru Y, Vuppusetty C, Wada H, et al. A protein deacetylase SIRT1 is a negative regulator of metalloproteinase-9. The FASEB Journal. 2009;**23**(9):2810-2819

[30] Rajendrasozhan S, Yang SR, Kinnula VL, Rahman I. SIRT1, an antiinflammatory and antiaging protein, is decreased in lungs of patients with chronic obstructive pulmonary disease. American Journal of Respiratory and Critical Care Medicine. 2008;**177**(8):861-870

[31] Baker JR, Vuppusetty C, Colley T, Papaioannou AI, Fenwick P, Donnelly L, Ito K, Barnes PJ. Oxidative stress dependent microRNA-34a activation via PI3Kα reduces the expression of sirtuin-1 and sirtuin-6 in epithelial cells. Scientific Reports. 2016 Oct 21;**6**:35871. DOI: 10.1038/srep35871

[32] Takasaka N, Araya J, Hara H, et al. Autophagy induction by SIRT6 through attenuation of insulin-like growth factor signaling is involved in the regulation of human bronchial epithelial cell senescence. Journal of Immunology. 2014;**192**(3):958-968

[33] Knobloch J, Wahl C, Feldmann M, Jungck D, Strauch J, Stoelben E, Koch A. Resveratrol attenuates the release of inflammatory cytokines from human bronchial smooth muscle cells exposed to lipoteichoic acid in chronic obstructive pulmonary disease. Basic & Clinical Pharmacology & Toxicology. 2014 Feb;**114**(2):202-209

[34] Malhotra R, Kurian N, Zhou XH, Jiang F, Monkley S, DeMicco A, Clausen IG, Delgren G, Edenro G, Ahdesmäki MJ, Clausen M, Öberg L, Israelsson E, Belfield G, Vaarala O. Altered regulation and expression of genes by BET family of proteins in COPD patients. PLoS One. 2017 Mar 1;**12**(3):e0173115. DOI: 10.1371/journal.pone.0173115 eCollection 2017. Erratum in: PLoS One. 2017 Apr 12;**12**(4):e0175997

[35] Nimmo ER, Prendergast JG, Aldhous MC, et al. Genome-wide methylation profiling in Crohn's disease identifies altered epigenetic regulation of key host defense mechanisms including the Th17 pathway. Inflammatory Bowel Diseases. 2012;**18**:889-899

[36] Nicodeme E, Jeffrey KL, Schaefer U, Beinke S, Dewell S, Chung C, et al. Suppression of inflammation by a synthetic histone mimic. Nature. 2010;**468**:1119-1123

[37] Ambros V. The functions of animal microRNAs. Nature. 2004;**431**:350-355

[38] De Flora S, Balansky R, D'Agostini F, et al. Smoke-induced microRNA and related proteome alterations. Modulation by chemopreventive agents. International Journal of Cancer. 2012;**131**(12):2763-2773

[39] Graff JW, Powers LS, Dickson AM, et al. Cigarette smoking decreases global microRNA expression in human alveolar macrophages. PLoS One. 2012;**7**(8):e44066

[40] Ezzie ME, Crawford M, Cho JH, et al. Gene expression networks in COPD: microRNA and mRNA regulation. Thorax. 2012;**67**(2):122-131

[41] Christenson SA, Brandsma CA, Campbell JD, et al. miR-638 regulates gene expression networks associated with emphysematous lung destruction. Genome Medicine. 2013;**5**(12):114

[42] Leidinger P, Keller A, Borries A, et al. Specific peripheral miRNA profiles for distinguishing lung cancer from COPD. Lung Cancer. 2011;**74**(1):41-47

[43] Sanfiorenzo C, Ilie MI, Belaid A, et al. Two panels of plasma microRNAs as non-invasive biomarkers for prediction of recurrence in resectable NSCLC. PLoS One. 2013;**8**(1):e54596

[44] Chatila WM, Criner GJ, Hancock WW, Akimova T, Moldover B, Chang JK, Cornwell W, Santerre M, Rogers TJ. Blunted expression of miR-199a-5p in regulatory T cells of patients with chronic obstructive pulmonary disease compared to unaffected smokers. Clinical and Experimental Immunology. 2014 Jul;**177**(1):341-352

Chapter 3

The Respiratory Microbiome in COPD

Orla O'Carroll, Joanna Peart, Eamon Mullen and
Conor Burke

Additional information is available at the end of the chapter

http://dx.doi.org/10.5772/intechopen.70776

Abstract

In classical teaching, the lungs were thought of as a sterile environment with the isolation of bacteria on sputum or bronchoalveolar lavage sampling felt to represent pathogenic colonisation in disease states. This teaching has been over-turned with the discovery of a rich microbiome in the respiratory tract. The respiratory microbiome is a huge target for novel research in many fields, most notable in that of airway diseases such as asthma and chronic obstructive pulmonary disease (COPD). Next-generation sequencing is a culture-independent method for microbial sampling which has transformed the accuracy and speed at which whole microbial communities can be described in studies. This has led to an explosion of knowledge regarding the human respiratory microbiome. COPD is a common, chronic disease of the respiratory system involving an irreversible airway obstruction which places huge burden on patients and healthcare systems alike. The respiratory microbiome is different in those who suffer from COPD than in those without the disease, but little is known as to the role of the microbiome in disease pathogenesis or manifestation. This chapter aims to outline the advances in sequencing methods in relation to the microbiome and establish a description of the respiratory microbiome in health and in COPD. We will describe the existing literature on the topic and discuss potential key areas for future research.

Keywords: microbiome, immune system, infection

1. Introduction

Chronic obstructive pulmonary disease (COPD) is a common, chronic respiratory disorder which affects millions of people worldwide [1]. It causes significant morbidity and mortality and poses a huge burden on healthcare systems through recurrent hospital admissions. Indeed, it was the fifth leading cause of death worldwide in 2002 and is estimated by the WHO to become the third leading cause of death internationally by 2030 [2]. In essence, COPD is characterised by an obstructive ventilatory deficit that is rarely reversible. Pathogenesis of the disease is most strongly associated with smoking though, certainly, there are other factors which can contribute to its development. Despite the ever-increasing prevalence of COPD worldwide, the exact roles of various causative factors and underlying disease mechanisms are not fully understood.

One such potential causative factor is the human microbiome, the collection of all the genomes of microorganisms living in association with the human body both in health and disease. The microbiota is composed of bacteria, fungi, viruses, protozoa and archaea (single-cell organisms). Microbial cells in humans are estimated to outweigh human cells by a ratio of 10 to 1, and microbial genes outweigh human genes by a factor of between 100 and 1000 [3]. Therefore, unsurprisingly, the microbiome has been implicated in many diseases across varied body systems including arthritis, colorectal cancer and inflammatory bowel disease [4, 5]. However, more recently attention has been paid to the role of the human microbiome in chronic respiratory diseases such as asthma, cystic fibrosis and COPD.

This chapter aims to explore the meaning of the microbiome and how it came to be such a current and relevant topic for high-level investigative research in the area of respiratory disease. We aim to review the existing literature on the topic and particularly explore the relationship between the microbiome and COPD exacerbation in terms of both infective and non-infective events. We will discuss the perceived importance of the gut microbiome with reference to respiratory health and disease and pay particular attention to the so-called gut-lung axis. Finally, we will discuss some potential topics for novel research in the field of microbiome analysis and discuss future directions for research.

2. The human microbiome: technological advances

Recent advances in next-generation sequencing technologies have caused a quantum leap in the analysis of microbial species in various body systems. The cornerstone of these technologies involves extraction, replication, and identification of specific highly conserved genes which are reproducible across a whole host of microbes. Total DNA is extracted from the given sample type, e.g., bronchoalveolar lavage, tissue biopsy samples, etc., and specific genes are polymerase chain reaction (PCR)-amplified using universal PCR primers to create amplicons. For bacteria, DNA coding for the 16S rRNA gene can be amplified and contains both variable sequence regions V1–V9 and the aforementioned highly conserved region present in all prokaryotes. 18S rRNA/internal transcribed spacer (ITS) genes are amplified and assessed for fungi and protozoa. The 18S rRNA gene is the conserved gene across these species, and analysis can be coupled with variable internal transcribed spacer (ITS) regions in order to achieve interspecies separation. Amplicons are then analysed using next-generation sequencing which allows rapid, simultaneous analysis, with sequences thus clustered into operational taxonomic units (OTUs). OTUs are then identified to the level of species, family or genus, by analysis against a reference database. In this way, microbial species can be rapidly and reliably identified in a culture-independent manner. Further to this, relative abundance of species in a given sample can be calculated to establish the richness and evenness of the microbiome in a system. This advance in technology has been responsible for the identification of the components of the gut microbiome in health, and much research on the microbiome of other systems has begun from this point [6].

There are a few key limitations involved in 16S rRNA and 18S rRNA/ITS gene sequencing methods for identification of bacterial and fungal species. Both techniques rely on the availability of highly specific, non-biased PCR primers as well as rich and varied reference libraries. The quality of PCR primers and references is generally held to be very high in the case of bacterial 16S rRNA sequencing [7] but less so in the case of fungal sequencing. Furthermore, little information is gained from both these methods about the biological function of these microbes. Despite this, they are considered to be cost-effective methods for assessing microbial diversity in a given sample.

Whole-genome shotgun sequencing is an advance on the above techniques whereby long DNA strands can be sequenced and identified rapidly. DNA strands are sheared into random fragments and cloned into a vector, historically *E. coli*. Clones are then sequenced to produce reads, and reads in turn are assembled into the original sequence using software programmes. This technique not only identifies microbes but can also infer information regarding biological function encoded in the whole genome. However, due to the massive amounts of complex DNA data processed, and the long reads that tend to be generated from this method, the system is open to errors. This is also a far more expensive method for DNA sequencing.

Next-generation sequencing employs similar methods to shotgun sequencing but generates hundreds of thousands of shorter reads in a smaller timeframe. This term is synonymous with high-throughput sequencing and encompasses multiple fast, effective, accurate sequencing methods. Some potential limitations include the presence of host DNA in the original sample, high costs of these methods and some difficulty drawing meaningful conclusions from vast quantities of extremely complex data.

Both 16S rRNA sequencing and next-generation sequencing are in use in laboratories worldwide, and both contribute to the advancement of our understanding of the microbiome through quick and accurate analysis of samples. As these technologies continue to advance and become more refined, they will become more affordable and sophisticated in coming years, allowing accessible DNA sequencing to come to the fore. Further analysis of RNA r and proteins can be achieved through the techniques of metatranscriptomics and metaproteomics, and this can give us information about genes and pathways in the context of microbiome sampling. See **Table 1** for a summary of terms relating to the various DNA sequencing techniques we have discussed above.

Term	Description
Microbiota	The collection of all microorganisms living in association with the human body or a specific system/environment
Microbiome	The genome of the human microbiota
Taxonomy	Classification system of organisms
Operational taxonomic unit	Categorisation of organisms into species by DNA sequence data
Metagenome	The collection of all genes obtained from microorganisms in a habitat
Next-generation sequencing	A collective term to describe high-throughput technologies. These allow rapid parallel DNA sequencing, i.e. Illumina (Solexa) sequencing, SOLiD sequencing
16S ribosomal gene	Gene encoding a 16S subunit of bacterial ribosomes that is highly conserved between different bacterial species
16SrRNA gene sequencing	Determining the DNA sequence of a 16S ribosomal gene
Metatranscriptomics	Analysis of mRNA transcripts associated with an organism
Metaproteomics	Analysis of microbial proteins
Metabolomics	Analysis of the set of metabolites present within an organism
Richness	The number of unique taxonomic units in a sample
Evenness	The relative number of taxonomic units in a sample
Alpha diversity	A measure of the richness and evenness in a sample
Beta diversity	A measure of the similarity of the bacterial composition between samples

Table 1. Summary of terms relating to DNA sequencing techniques.

3. The respiratory microbiome

For a long time, the respiratory system was thought of as a fully sterile environment. Culture isolates from sputum and bronchoalveolar lavage samples were felt to exclusively represent pathogenic colonisation in disease states and exacerbation. However, this classic teaching was challenged, only in 2009, with the publication of a study undertaken by Hilty et al. [8] which employed 16S rRNA sequencing techniques to analyse the microbiota of the lower respiratory tract. Subjects carried either a diagnosis of asthma or COPD or were healthy controls, and all underwent bronchoscopy to obtain endobronchial brushings from the left upper lobe. The microbiome of the nasal cavity and oropharynx was also sampled using surface swabs. This study found a similar abundance of microbes in all groups (with a range of 1–10 million cells per sample) but with significant differences in microbial composition between the groups studied. This was the first study of its kind and was understandably met with scepticism as it challenged the formal teaching on the subject [9]. Critics were quick to point out limitations of the study design including the fact that lower airway sampling could easily be confounded by passage of the bronchoscope through the upper airways, the oropharynx having a significantly higher bacterial load than the lower respiratory tract in the order of 1–10 billion cells per sample. Additionally, it was felt that the relatively new (at the time) process of 16S rRNA sequencing would identify dead bacteria in most of the samples and that in order to address this potential confounder, a stronger control group was needed. Nevertheless this was an interesting and well-designed starting point for the explosion of interest in the area that was to follow.

A follow-up study which was similar in design and conducted in 'healthy smokers', and patients with COPD confirmed the presence of microbial colonies in the lower respiratory tract but again was open to the aforementioned potential confounders [10]. These confounders were first addressed by Charlson et al. [9] in 2011 who designed a study using double bronchoscopy in six healthy individuals. This involved a process of initial bronchoscopy to anaesthetise the airway and then the use of an uncontaminated bronchoscope to collect samples by brush and lavage. To further reduce the confounding potential of the environment on the scope, saline washes were used before the scope was inserted, and this saline was analysed for bacterial load. Microbiota was found to be present in all lower respiratory samples from all patients, but unlike the previously mentioned studies, the order of magnitude was far lower, 100–1000 cells per sample. The investigators performed serial lavage, results of which showed sequentially diminishing bacterial load. They inferred from this that there is marked carry-over from the upper to the lower respiratory tracts. An interesting finding was that low levels of DNA were found in the environmental control samples such as the saline washes even though these were sterile by culture. Bacterial lines were found to be more abundant in the lower airway than the upper, though overall microbiome was more rich in the upper airway.

The Hilty trial found that the bronchial tree consists of a rich and varied microbial community in all groups tested and confirmed that the individual components of this community were different in health and disease [8]. *Proteobacteria* were found in higher abundance in diseased individuals (those with asthma and COPD) than in controls, in particular the well-known respiratory pathogens *Haemophilus, Moraxella* and *Neisseria.* In contrast, *Bacteroidetes* such as *Prevotella* were found to be far more abundant in healthy controls. Studies since this have aimed to further refine our understanding of the now-accepted paradigm of the core respiratory microbiome. Various studies have identified varying counts of microbes, and it is generally acknowledged that the respiratory microbiome is composed of *Bacteroides, Proteobacteriae, Firmicutes* and *Actinobacteriae.* The bacterial communities of the lung are almost mirrored in the oral cavity, but not in the nose, and some species that show high prevalence in the mouth become less abundant lower in the lungs. This has led some to believe that oral microbes which migrate to the lower respiratory tract can be selectively eliminated from healthy lungs and that those which are not eliminated may contribute to low-level inflammatory processes [11].

These studies and numerous similar trials [12, 13] have established the existence of the respiratory microbiome. As technology improves, our ability to sample and analyse these complex microbial communities will continue to expand until we have a full understanding of not only the composition but also the function of the human respiratory microbiome.

4. Establishment of the microbiome and the relationship between microbiota and the immune system

We have discussed the basis of our understanding thus far of the existence of the microbiome in the lung and will go on to explore the role of the microbiome in health and disease. However we must first try to decipher the way in which the microbiome is established in humans in order to assess whether differences in development may confer lasting effects on the microbiome in later life. It has long been believed that exposure to various bacteria in youth may alter the way disease manifests in later life. The so-called hygiene hypothesis states that reduced exposure to microorganisms in infancy increases a person's likelihood to develop allergic-type diseases by suppressing the natural development of the immune system, particularly the innate immune response. It would therefore follow that interruptions in the natural development of the microbiome could confer long-lasting differences in the respiratory microbiome and that this may have knock-on effects to an individual's immunity and their propensity to develop certain diseases. Much of what is known about the development of the microbiome comes from studies of gut microbiota, and we will explore some of this literature in this section in order to assess potential links between the microbiome and immune system dysfunction.

Gut microbiota has an established role in the development and maturation of the immune response via the so-called education of mucosal surfaces and systemic immune response systems. Studies suggest that there is a critical development time between months 12 and 24 in the relationship between the gut microbiome and the building of the immune system [14]. This is demonstrated by the increased risk of the development of inflammatory autoimmune disease where dysbiosis is caused by the use of antibiotics at a critical time in infancy. For example, increased rates of immunologic disorders such as asthma and paediatric irritable bowel disease are associated with antibiotic use in infancy [15].

Traditionally, the human gut has been assumed to be sterile at birth. However, recent advances in PCR techniques as outlined above have found evidence of bacteria consistent with the maternal gut microbiota in meconium. This is believed to have been transferred via the maternal blood stream [16]. Further exposure is from diet and the surrounding environment, including the birth canal. Indeed, even the mode of delivery at birth can confer lasting changes on the developing microbiome, with those born via caesarean section found to have significantly lower abundance and diversity of gut *Bacteroides* and *Actinobacteria* species in the first 3 months of life [17]. At age 12 and 24 months, the infant gut resembles that of the adult [18]. The gut microbiome is relatively stable until late in life and has the ability to restore itself [19].

Evidence supports reduced childhood morbidity and mortality not only during the period of lactation but also beyond this period and into adulthood [20]. Facultative anaerobes create an anaerobic environment where obligate anaerobic bacteria such as *Bifidobacterium* species flourish. *Bifidobacteria* dominate the gut microbiota, and milk oligosaccharides are known to stimulate their proliferation [16]. Along with *lactobacilli* they appear to maintain resistance to pathogenic colonisation, in short acting as so-termed good bugs. *Bifidobacteria* are rarely pathogenic and ferment bacteria to produce short-chain fatty acids (SCFA) [16].

SCFAs are thought to have many functions including important interactions with the immune system. Two mechanisms of action for this relationship have been established to date, activation of G-protein-coupled receptors (GPR41 and GPR43) and inhibition of histone deacetylase (HDAC) via leukocytes and endothelial cell lines. SCFAs also have a regulatory role over leukocyte functions such as production of cytokines (TNF-α, IL-2, IL-6 and IL-10), eicosanoids and chemokines. In addition, SCFAs also seem to impact the migratory ability of leukocytes to travel to points of inflammation and to destroy microbial pathogens [21].

Intestinal epithelial cells are a key component of the symbiotic relationship between gut microbiota and the host. They provide a physical and chemical barrier system to spatially separate gut microbiota from the host immune system, preventing unnecessary immune responses. Immunological mediators such as cytokines and chemokines are secreted from intestinal epithelial cells which are in turn stimulated by gut microbiota-modulated host immune responses, maintaining a well-balanced relationship between gut microbes and the host immune system [22]. Gut microbiota also have a role in the maintenance of innate immunity. For example, murein lipoprotein from selective gut-symbiotic Gram-negative bacteria results in IgG targeting bacterial antigens for removal by phagocytes [23].

In addition, gut microbiota plays an important role in the development of both local and remote adaptive immunities as demonstrated by the work with germ-free (GF) mice which had significantly lower numbers of CD4+ cells. In other animal model research, the spleens and mesenteric lymph nodes of GF animals were shown to have abnormalities such as absent lymphocyte zones. Th1/Th2 imbalances have also been demonstrated in GF animal models [24].

New techniques have allowed even specific bacterial species to be associated with the development of particular T-cell subtypes. For example, *Bacteroides fragilis* is involved in the induction of the development of a systemic Th1 response via its polysaccharide A (PSA) molecules [21].

There seems to be emerging evidence to suggest a significant relationship between the gut microbiome and the respiratory microbiome proposing the existence of a 'lung-gut axis'. When depletion of gut microbiota is achieved in mouse models, the mice are prone to developing significant pneumonia, and when the gut microbiome is restored, the severity of pneumonia decreases [25]. Additionally, this relationship is strengthened by the observation that acute changes in the gut microbiota can be achieved by stimulation of the lung with lipopolysaccharide [26]. These results indicate the potential for 'cross-talk' between the gut and the lung and introduce the concept of a 'whole body microbiome', dysregulation of which can lead to disease in other organ systems.

As we can see, mostly from gut microbiome research trials, there is significant interplay between the microbial communities in the gut and the immune system, both adaptive and innate immune responses. The microbiome is established in a well-described manner but can certainly be greatly influenced by diet, microbial exposures, and even mode of delivery at birth. It is reasonable to expect the same interplay to be a feature of the respiratory microbiome, but further work is needed to establish this relationship.

5. The microbiome in stable COPD

We have explored the current knowledge of the respiratory microbiome in health and the role it plays in inflammatory processes; however, we will now discuss what is known about the role of the respiratory microbiome in relation to COPD. *Haemophilus influenzae, Moraxella catarrhalis* and *Streptococcus pneumoniae* are known to be the most abundant colonisers in the lungs of COPD patients [27]. Consequently, they are the most frequently isolated pathogens in sputum samples and bronchoalveolar lavage in this patient group, both in health and disease. These microbes remain prominent across multiple studies of the COPD lung and are implicated in driving multiple inflammatory pathways in the diseased lung [28, 29]. This certainly has many profound clinical effects on patient groups with COPD. For example, a recent study found that patients who were chronically colonised with *H. influenzae* were more likely to have increased airway inflammation and decreased lung volumes when compared with those not colonised [30].

In healthy lungs, spatial and temporal microbial diversity in the same lung is less than the diversity seen between individuals and seems to be mostly a consequence of microbial elimination and immigration. The reverse is true in diseased lungs meaning there is wide variation in microbial communities in a given patient's lungs [31]. This is particularly true of COPD lungs where very significant temporal and biogeographical variations in diversity and abundance have been seen [32]. Microbial communities are felt to be drastically affected by local growth conditions in disease lung. The factors which can affect growth conditions are oxygen tension, pH, relative number of immune cells present in a given area and even blood perfusion. The microbiome has been linked to the clinical phenotype of COPD by one group who concluded that greater emphysema and increased immune cell infiltration were found in those COPD patients who showed decline in the diversity and richness of their respiratory microbiome [12]. Indeed more recently, correlation was shown between altered bacterial communities as seen in COPD with CT-detectable structural changes in lungs of those COPD patients [33].

Reactive oxygen species are postulated to drive the inflammatory processes which lead to COPD through activated alveolar macrophages. Bacterial activation of certain NOD-like receptors can upregulate the production of these reactive oxygen species in alveolar macrophages. Bacterial activation such as this is known to occur in the GI tract, and this potentially implicates the GI microbiota in the development of COPD [34]. If gut microbiome can potentially be implicated in driving respiratory inflammation, it is reasonable to wonder whether the use of certain probiotic bacterial strains could help to reduced lung-driven inflammatory processed. One group has shown favourable outcomes with regard to this hypothesis and has found that when alveolar macrophages phagocytose the well-known probiotic strains *Lactobacillus rhamnosus* and *Bifidobacterium breve*, certain inflammatory pathways are suppressed. In particular their use inhibits cigarette smoke-induced nuclear factor-kB activation and the inflammation associated with this pathway [35].

6. The impact of the microbiome on infection and exacerbation

As we have discussed, there is an increasing wealth of evidence indicating the vital role that the lung microbiome plays in chronic obstructive pulmonary disease (COPD); however, our understanding of the exact role the lung microbiome plays in COPD exacerbation remains in its infancy. While our understanding of the microbiome in humans has vastly expanded in recent years, there is still a significant dearth of certainty regarding the dynamics of the lung microbiome and its role in disease aetiology. Ambiguity arises from the heterogeneous nature of COPD coupled with the diversity and structure of the microbiome, the mediation of host inflammatory response and additional external variables such as involvement of antibiotic and steroid treatments and environmental factors.

Recent literature contributions have highlighted the central and crucial role of bacteria in COPD exacerbations with evidence to suggest that during exacerbations there is a shift in microbial diversity within the ecosystem. [36]. An increase in the relative abundance of *Proteobacteria* and a decrease in *Firmicutes* compared to non-exacerbation samples have been observed. Interestingly, there is an increase in *Moraxella* and *Haemophilus* populations during exacerbations with a concurrent decrease in *Streptococcus* identified. These shifts in taxa composition are in keeping with the findings of Wang et al. [37] who found an overall reduction in alpha diversity, the microbial diversity within a sample, during exacerbations when compared with 'stable' samples.

Network analysis has revealed potential interactions between bacterial operational taxonomic units (OTUs). Microbial network examination has revealed that a few 'hub' OTUs predominate which are highly connected with multiple other nodes of microbiota. Moreover, many of the OTUs demonstrate both 'coexistence' and 'co-exclusion' patterns between bacterial species. Most OTUs have numerous negative connections with other members of the microbiota. In particular, *Haemophilus* has a disproportionately large number of negative connections with other OTUs [38]. Consequently, any significant increase in abundance of OTUs is associated with a decrease in microbial alpha diversity. Conversely many OTUs demonstrate a strong mutual cooperative relationship in tightly connected groups. Indeed, a 'Like Will to Like' relationship of enrichment promotion among organisms of different species in an ecosystem has been well described for intestinal microbiota [39], whereby closely related phylotypes display significantly increased abundances or co-occurrences when compared with those less closely related species.

In the context of the lung microbiome, the keystone species is a topic that warrants further exploration. This inchoate paradigm, which expounds the concept describing how minimal fluctuations in the abundances of relatively few bacterial species may profoundly alter the microbial community dynamic and potentially impact the human disease state [37]. For example, *Actinobacteria,* a species whose abundance decreases during COPD exacerbations, comprises a multitude of metabolically diverse organisms which produce secondary metabolites, including those with antimicrobial activity [40]. Moreover, many *Clostridia* species are known activators of anti-inflammatory T-regulatory cells [41].

Following on, it is possible that the overgrowth of certain OTUs may drive dysbiosis of the respiratory tract through remodelling of the normal lung microbial ecosystem which could elicit a host pro-inflammatory response [37]. Through dysbiosis of the lung microbiota, pathogenic members of the genera *Haemophilus* and *Moraxella* can indirectly trigger excessive production of chemokine ligand 8/interleukin 8 (CXCL8/IL-8). This is due to pathogenic *Haemophilus* and *Moraxella* members directly causing inflammation by exposing the host to lipopolysaccharides and other pathogen-associated molecular patterns [41]. This is coupled with depletion of species that might in fact contribute to the maintenance of community and host immune homeostasis and fight the negative effects of the above pathogenic species.

As a corollary, one potential biomarker for overall microbial lung population is sputum CXCL8/IL-8, which is directly associated with microbiome community structure and diversity. It has a prominent role in COPD [42] whereby it induces airway inflammation by recruiting neutrophils and upregulating mucin genes, causing mucus production. As such, sputum CXCl8/IL-8 levels correlate well with COPD severity [43].

Given the heterogeneous nature of COPD, identification of various phenotypes has helped in identifying the most suitable and specific treatment for exacerbations. The microbiome exacerbation phenotypes have been defined as bacterial, viral, eosinophilic, bacterial/viral combination, bacterial/eosinophilic combination or pauci-inflammatory [36]. There is a significant difference in microbiome composition at both the phylum and genus levels between different phenotypes but particularly between bacterial and eosinophilic exacerbations. Furthermore, there is a significant decrease in the *Proteobacteria/Firmicutes* ratio in the eosinophilic subgroup, compared to the other phenotypes, during exacerbations. This correlates with the hypothesis that exacerbations involving bacteria and eosinophils reflect fundamental differences in their immunopathogenesis, while virus-related exacerbations are often associated with both bacterial infections and an increase of eosinophils [36]. Consequently, the presence or absence of eosinophilic inflammation could therefore potentially be used as a biomarker for stratification of the underlying associated microbiome and subsequent treatment strategies.

With regard to COPD exacerbation treatment strategies, it has become apparent that 'standard-of-care' therapy involving antibiotics and steroids has a significant effect on the phylogenetic composition of the community. Alterations in the abundance of individual taxa are directly linked to the use of steroids and/or antibiotics. Indeed, the use of oral corticosteroids has been found to decrease microbial alpha diversity, with an enrichment of some taxa, mainly *Proteobacteria*, and an increase in the *Proteobacteria/Firmicutes* ratio has been identified. In contrast, a reversal of this trend, i.e. an increase in microbial alpha diversity and microbial composition changes, has been observed when treatment of COPD exacerbation involves antibiotics (with or without steroids) [37, 43]. Furthermore, this effect of antibiotic and steroid treatment on the microbiome structure appears to be prolonged, emphasising the importance of patient phenotype stratification.

7. A functional analysis of COPD airway microbiome

A recently developed bioinformatics tool, PICRUSt [41, 44], has enabled researchers to explore the predicted functional capacity of the microbiota involved in the changes observed during exacerbation and response to treatment. Hitherto, high-resolution metagenomic profiling has been almost prohibitively expensive and intensive computationally. PICRUSt can predict the presence and relative abundance of gene families within the microbiome. This prediction is based on 16S rRNA data and can be used at any time point or, in this case, during an exacerbation. The intention is to identify and characterise variations in microbiome differential associated with features of exacerbations. Predicted functions that are enriched during exacerbation include pathways involved in apoptosis, p53 signalling, along with those involved in bacterial and viral infection, e.g. *Influenza A* virus and *Staphylococcus aureus*. On the other hand, depleted predicted functions include those pathways involved in the response to viral infection, e.g. RIG-I-like receptor signalling. Other known pathways depleted during COPD exacerbation include those involved in the production of betalain and indole alkaloid—known for their antimicrobial properties—and those involved in flavonoid and steroid biosynthesis, known anti-inflammatory mediators [41]. In keeping with this hypothesis, a reversal of the above compositional shifts in the microbiome can be observed during treatment and indeed may play a role in the recovery from exacerbation.

Observations suggest that while variation between test subjects in microbial community dynamics at exacerbation is seen, the compositional shifts overall for a particular microbiome are not very large. These finding suggests that exacerbations of COPD could result from the cumulative effects of many small-scale changes in the community composition. Hence, these functional predictions may describe not only an increase in pathogen-elicited inflammation but also the loss of crucial protective functions in the microbiome.

8. Conclusions and areas for future research

Throughout this chapter, we have outlined the relatively new field of microbiome analysis in respiratory disease. The lungs were once thought to be sterile, and since this presumption was first over-turned in 2009, there has been a veritable explosion in the wealth of knowledge surrounding the topic. We are now beginning to understand the vital role which the microbiome plays in the development and propagation of many major respiratory diseases. This increased knowledge has been made possible by significant advances in culture-independent sequencing methods which we have outlined. As these intricate systems continue to develop and improve, our ability to analyse microbial samples will continue to strengthen with these techniques becoming more and more widespread and accessible.

Much is known about the gut microbiome, with respiratory microbiome research also on the increase. We have outlined some emerging evidence to suggest interplay between these two large micro-systems, and the hypothesis that they can mutually influence each other in health and disease is a fascinating concept. Certainly, more work needs to be done in this area through observational human research, as most of the literature involves animal models.

We now are in the position to not only name the components of a given microbiome but also to analyse their functions through next-generation metagenomics sequencing. It is not enough to know that the microbiome of the lung is altered in COPD; we must follow on to assess the function of these different bacteria and viruses in causing or preventing disease. If we can manage to do this in a meaningful and reproducible way for certain diseases such as asthma and COPD, then it is reasonable to assume that we can develop novel therapeutic targets for these chronic disease states which may alleviate the treatment burden for our patients.

Author details

Orla O'Carroll*, Joanna Peart, Eamon Mullen and Conor Burke

*Address all correspondence to: oocarroll@gmail.com

Respiratory Department, James Connolly Memorial Hospital, Blanchardstown, Dublin, Ireland

References

[1] GBD 2015 Chronic Respiratory Disease Collaborators. Global, regional, and national deaths, prevalence, disability-adjusted life years, and years lived with disability for chronic obstructive pulmonary disease and asthma, 1990-2015: A systematic analysis for the global burden of disease study 2015. Lancet Respiratory Medicine. 2017 Aug 16; pii: S2213-2600(17)30293-X. Vol 5, No.9, p. 691-706

[2] World Health Organisation, Global Status Report on Noncommunicable Diseases 2010: Description of the Global Burden of NCDs their Risk Factors and Development. WHO Press. ISBN: 978 92 4156422 9

[3] Palm NW, de Zoete MR, Flavell RA. Immune–microbiota interactions in health and disease. Clinical Immunology. **159**(2):122-127

[4] Knights D, Lassen KG, Xavier RJ. Advances in inflammatory bowel disease pathogenesis: Linking host genetics and the microbiome. Gut. 2013;**62**(10):1505-1510

[5] Le Chatelier E, Nielsen T, Qin J, et al. Richness of human gut microbiome correlates with metabolic markers. Nature. 2013;**500**(7464):541-546

[6] Sharpton TJ. An introduction to the analysis of shotgun metagenomic data. Frontiers in Plant Science. 2014;**5**:1-14

[7] Anderson IC, Campbell CD, Prosser JI. Potential bias of fungal 18S rDNA and internal transcribed spacer polymerase chain reaction primers for estimating fungal biodiversity in soil. Environmental Microbiology. 2003;**5**:36-47

[8] Hilty M, Burke C, Pedro H, Cardenas P, Bush A, Bossley C, Davies J, Ervine A, Poulter L, Pachter L, et al. Disordered microbial communities in asthmatic airways. PLoS One. 2010;**5**:e8578

[9] Charlson ES, Bittinger K, Haas AR, Fitzgerald AS, Frank I, Yadav A, Bushman FD, Collman RG. Topographical continuity of bacterial populations in the healthy human respiratory tract. American Journal of Respiratory and Critical Care Medicine. 2011;**184**:957-963

[10] Erb-Downward JR, Thompson DL, Han MK, Freeman CM, McCloskey L, Schmidt LA, Young VB, Toews GB, Curtis JL, Sundaram B, et al. Analysis of the lung microbiome in the 'healthy' smoker and in COPD. PLoS One. 2011;**6**:e16384

[11] Larsen JM, Steen-Jensen DB, Laursen JM, Sondergaard JN, Musavian HS, Butt TM, et al. Divergent pro-inflammatory profile of human dendritic cells in response to commensal and pathogenic bacteria associated with the airway microbiota. PLoS One. 2012;**7**:e31976

[12] Sze MA, Dimitriu PA, Hayashi S, et al. The lung tissue microbiome in chronic obstructive pulmonary disease. American Journal of Respiratory and Critical Care Medicine. 2012;**185**(10):1073-1080

[13] Huang YJ, Kim E, Cox MJ, et al. A persistent and diverse airway microbiota present during chronic obstructive pulmonary disease exacerbations. OMICS Journal. 2010;**14**(1):9-59

[14] Martin R, Makino H, Cetinyurek Yavuz A, Ben-Amor K, Roelofs M, Ishikawa E, et al. Early-life events, including mode of delivery and type of feeding, siblings and gender, shape the developing gut microbiota. PLoS One. 2016;**11**:e0158498

[15] Shanahan F. The colonic microbiota in health and disease. Current Opinion in Gastroenterology. 2013 Jan;**29**(1):49-54

[16] Firmansyah A, Chongviriyaphan N, Dillon DH, Khan NC, Morita T, Tontisirin K, Tuyen LD, Wang W, Bindels J, Deurenberg P, Ong S, Hautvast J, Meyer D, Vaughan EE. Fructans in the first 1000 days of life and beyond, and for pregnancy. Asia Pacific Journal of Clinical Nutrition. 2016 Dec;**25**(4):652-675

[17] Rutayisire E, Huang K, Liu Y, Tao F. The mode of delivery affects the diversity and colonization pattern of the gut microbiota during the first year of infants' life: A systematic review. BMC Gastroenterology. 2016;**16**:1-12

[18] D'Aversa F, Tortora A, Ianiro G, Ponziani FR, Annicchiarico BE, Gasbarrini A. Gut microbiota and metabolic syndrome. Internal and Emergency Medicine. 2013 Apr;**8**(Suppl. 1): S11-S15. DOI: 10.1007/s11739-013-0916-z Review. PubMed PMID: 23468402

[19] Quigley E. Gut microbiota and the role of probiotics in therapy. Current Opinion in Pharmacology. 2011;**11**:593-603

[20] Cacho NT, Lawrence RM. Innate immunity and breast milk. Frontiers in Immunology. 2017;**8**:584

[21] Vinolo MAR et al. Regulation of inflammation by short chain fatty acids. Nutrients. 2011;**3**(10):858-876 PMC. Web. 18 July 2017

[22] Okumura R, Takeda K. Roles of intestinal epithelial cells in the maintenance of gut homeostasis. Experimental & Molecular Medicine. 2017;**49**(5):e338

[23] Shukla SD, Budden KF, Neal R, Hansbro PM. Microbiome effects on immunity, health and disease in the lung. Clinical & Translational Immunology. 2017 Mar 10;**6**(3):e133

[24] Wu H-J, Eric W. The role of gut microbiota in immune homeostasis and autoimmunity. Gut Microbes. 2012;**3**(1):4-14

[25] Schuijt TJ, Lankelma JM, Scicluna BP, De Sousa e Melo F, Roelofs JJ, de Boer JD, et al. The gut microbiota plays a protective role in the host defence against pneumococcal pneumonia. Gut. 2016;**65**:575-583.

[26] Sze MA, Tsuruta M, Yang SW, Oh Y, Man SF, et al. Changes in the bacterial microbiota in gut, blood, and lungs following acute LPS instillation into mice lungs. PLoS One. 2014;**9**:e111228

[27] Barker BL, Haldar K, Patel H, Pavord ID, Barer MR, Brightling CE, et al. Association between pathogens detected using quantitative polymerase chain reaction with airway inflammation in COPD at stable state and exacerbations. Chest. 2015;**147**:46-55

[28] Simpson JL, Baines KJ, Horvat JC, Essilfie AT, Brown AC, Tooze M, et al. COPD is characterized by increased detection of *Haemophilus influenzae, Streptococcus pneumoniae* and a deficiency of bacillus species. Respirology. 2016;**21**:697-704

[29] Tay HL, Kaiko GE, Plank M, Li J, Maltby S, Essilfie AT, et al. Antagonism of miR-328 increases the antimicrobial function of macrophages and neutrophils and rapid clearance of non-typeable *Haemophilus influenzae* (NTHi) from infected lung. PLoS Pathogens. 2015;**11**:e1004549

[30] Tufvesson E, Bjermer L, Ekberg M. Patients with chronic obstructive pulmonary disease and chronically colonized with *Haemophilus influenzae* during stable disease phase have increased airway inflammation. International Journal of Chronic Obstructive Pulmonary Disease. 2015;**10**:881-889

[31] Dickson RP, Erb-Downward JR, Freeman CM, McCloskey L, Beck JM, Huffnagle GB, et al. Spatial variation in the healthy human lung microbiome and the adapted island model of lung biogeography. Annals of the American Thoracic Society. 2015;**12**:821-830

[32] Pragman AA, Kim HB, Reilly CS, Wendt C, Isaacson RE. The lung microbiome in moderate and severe chronic obstructive pulmonary disease. PLoS One. 2012;**7**:e47305

[33] Engel M, Endesfelder D, Schloter-Hai B, et al. Influence of lung CT changes in chronic obstructive pulmonary disease (COPD) on the human lung microbiome. PLoS One. 2017;**12**(7):e0180859

[34] Clarke TB. Early innate immunity to bacterial infection in the lung is regulated systemically by the commensal microbiota via nod-like receptor ligands. Infection and Immunity. 2014;**82**:4596-4606

[35] Mortaz E, Adcock IM, Ricciardolo FL, Varahram M, Jamaati H, Velayati AA, et al. Anti-inflammatory effects of *Lactobacillus rhamnosus* and *Bifidobacterium breve* on cigarette smoke activated human macrophages. PLoS One. 2015;**10**:e0136455

[36] Chambers DC et al. JTD special edition 'hot topics in COPD'—The microbiome in COPD. Journal of Thoracic Disease. 2014;**6**(11):1525-1531

[37] Wang Z, Bafadhel M, Haldar K, et al. Lung microbiome dynamics in COPD exacerbations. The European Respiratory Journal. 2016 Apr;**47**(4):1082-1092

[38] Mell JC, Hall IM, Redfield RJ. Defining the DNA uptake specificity of naturally competent *Haemophilus Influenzae* cells. Nucleic Acids Research. 2012;**40**(17):8536-8549 PMC. Web. 29 Aug 2017

[39] Stecher B, Chaffron S, Käppeli R, Hapfelmeier S, Freedrich S, Weber TC, et al. Like will to like: Abundances of closely related species can predict susceptibility to intestinal colonization by pathogenic and commensal bacteria. PLoS Pathogens. 2010;**6**(1):e1000711. DOI: https://doi.org/10.1371/journal.ppat.1000711

[40] Huang YJ, Boushey HA. The sputum microbiome in chronic obstructive pulmonary disease exacerbations. Annals of the American Thoracic Society. 2015;**12**(Suppl 2):S176-S180 PMC. Web. 20 July 2017

[41] Huang YJ et al. Airway microbiome dynamics in exacerbations of chronic obstructive pulmonary disease. Gilligan PH, editor. Journal of Clinical Microbiology. 2014;**52**(8): 2813-2823

[42] Mukaida N. Pathophysiological roles of interleukin-8/CXCL8 in pulmonary diseases. American Journal of Physiology – Lung Cellular and Molecular Physiology. Apr 2003; **284**(4):L566-L577

[43] Lee KY, Ho SC, Wang CH, et al. Reduced nuclear factor-kB repressing factor: A link toward systemic inflammation in COPD. The European Respiratory Journal. 2012 Oct;**40**(4):863-873

[44] Millares L et al. Functional metagenomics of the bronchial microbiome in COPD. PLoS One. 2015;**10**(12):e0144448

Chapter 4

Neurocognitive Impairment as Systemic Effects of COPD

Cristian Oancea, Emanuela Tudorache and
Voicu Tudorache

Additional information is available at the end of the chapter

http://dx.doi.org/10.5772/intechopen.70580

Abstract

Mild cognitive impairment (MCI), also known as incipient dementia, is characterized by the decline of cognitive function greater than expected for a certain age and educational level of the individual but not severe enough to interfere with their daily activities. However, this mild cognitive impairment affects several areas: visuospatial, memory, attention and fluency and it is a significant concern because it decreases the quality of life and treatment adherence of these patients. On the other hand, evidence suggests that individuals with Chronic obstructive pulmonary disease (COPD) also present an important risk of falls: 46% of these patients experience a fall/year, sometimes with fatal consequences. Standard clinical balance measures can predict the risk of falls in this population. Moreover, increased inflammatory biomarkers are associated with the decrease of cognitive functions and a higher risk of falls in this population. Patients with COPD have a higher balance and cognitive impairment than their healthy peers Therefore, it is important to identify, assess and understand the relevance of these comorbidities in order to characterize the full clinical spectrum of COPD and adjust prevention strategies, given the devastating consequences of these problems.

Keywords: balance, falls, dementia, cognition, COPD

1. Introduction

COPD is recognized as a disease with many systemic components [1]. Among them, the neuro-psychical component (anxiety/depression), has already been recognized. Besides this, in the last decade, research has been initiated on the neuromorphological substrate to explain whether certain manifestations such as cognition alteration, the occurrence of balance disorders, etc. could also be due to the impact of COPD, or would only be manifestations related to age and/or other comorbidities. This paper presents an overview of the state of knowledge in this last field.

1.1. Summary

- Cognition – domain and modulating factors.
- Balance disorders: nosology, prevalence, clinical consequences.
- COPD: fundamental pathophysiological mechanisms susceptible to alter cerebral function.
- Clinical consequences of affected cognition; measure methods.
- Therapeutic implications; preventive strategies.

2. Cognition: domain and modulating factors

There are multiple classifications of cognition, of which that proposed by Dal Negro seems the most appropriate for the purpose of this chapter. According to that, its domains and subdomains are: (a) executional function with the subdomains: attention, problem solving, planning and reasoning; (b) language, with the subdomains: comprehension and verbal fluency; (c) memory, with the subdomains: memory-based tagging and work memory; (d) praxis, with the subdomains: motor-ideative, ideative and visual constructive [2].

The distinction between any cognitive impairment and mild cognitive impairment (MCI) should be clarified. The latter refers to a brain function syndrome involving the onset and evolution of cognitive impairments other than those age and education related, but that are not significant enough to interfere with daily activities [3]. To date (2017), one of the most comprehensive meta-analyses that have specifically investigated prevalence MCI in the context of COPD, included 23,116 people with COPD, and showed MCI prevalence of 25%, raising up to 32% if any cognitive impairment is assessed [4].

Compared to the prevalence of MCI in the general population, which is in the range of 10–20% in older adults, a rate of 25–32% present in patients with COPD is more than worrying [5].

But equally important is the relationship between the various cognitive domains affected in COPD patients and the disease itself. This is because the prevalence of impairment varies among the different cognitive domains. What is more, the psychometric profile impairment would be associated with the variable components of COPD such as hypoxemia, hypercapnia, lung function, exacerbations or disease severity.

Although one cannot speak about a specific profile encountered in "pure" COPD, that is, the one without comorbidities, the most frequently affected subdomains are attention, naming, visuospatial, memory, motor and executive function and mood decrements (fear and antinociception) [6–10].

We must be aware that COPD severity (hypoxemia/hypercapnia, pulmonary obstruction and exacerbations), factors typically present (age and smoking) as well as various combinations (comorbidities, education level, physical activity, nutritional status, etc.) make up in a complex mosaic. Assigning cognition alterations to the underlying disease (COPD), implies for this reason, an extremely laborious and unlikely effort to distinguish among these factors. An example, in a prospective study of 62 patients with COPD, it was possible to see how cognitive impairment varied depending on the stage of the disease: exacerbation, at discharge or when the stable phase was reached; unlike other studies, this research followed the same patient at all 3 different stages of his disease. Cognitive assessment was measured by Montreal cognitive assessment (MoCA) test. From exacerbation to stable COPD, all the clinical variables improved step-by-step: visual-constructional, attention, language, abstraction, delayed recall and orientation (from exacerbation to discharge), visual-constructional and naming (from discharge to stable phase) and taken as a whole, from exacerbation to stable COPD: naming, attention, language, abstraction and delayed recall [11].

Thus, differences in studies such as (a) various study designs and methodological limitations: lack of clinical assessment of airflow impairment, severity of COPD, heterogeneity of assessment moment (stable phase, exacerbation and long-term oxygen therapy [LTOT]), small sample size, lack of appropriate referent group, diagnostic criteria for cognitive impairment (psychometric tools and neuroimaging), (b) the use of different definition, (c) lack confounder adjustment procedures: comorbidities, age, active smokers, level of education, etc., may explain the wide range of prevalence rates of cognitive impairment in COPD from 5.5% up to 77% [12, 13].

2.1. Balance disorders: nosology, prevalence, clinical consequences

Chronic illnesses in general as the disease progresses develop debilitating features, and COPD is no exception. Age and other features may include lower limb muscle weakness, overall fatigue, dizziness, different functional impairment, body imbalance and others [14].

Among them we will refer to balance impairment, which can lead to the loss of coordination and implicitly to falls.

Involuntary falls are incidents that can occur at any age, more frequently in the elderly, with possible devastating consequences. Individuals aged over 65 would experience at least one fall per year [15]. In a prospective study, the incidence of falls was more than four times higher in patients with COPD, than in healthy individuals with respect to gender and age [16].

Due to comorbidities, elderly patients are often polymedicated: anxiolytics/sedatives, antihypertensives, corticosteroids, etc., medications that can be responsible for balance disturbances. According to a research conducted by Roig, the use of corticosteroid therapy in COPD population has been estimated to be ~61.5% for inhaled and ~8.3% for oral corticosteroids [17]. Corticosteroid therapy interferes with the production of contractile proteins (increase intracellular proteolysis) resulting in muscle weakness conducing to falls. Thus, in order to relate falls to COPD we must exclude other confounders: polypharmacy, decreased vision, impaired mobility (arthrosis) and multiple other comorbidities.

Two other factors, such as sedentary life style and systemic inflammation, should not be neglected either: the former is almost constantly encountered and the latter in about 30% of cases [18].

Severe COPD stages as well as exacerbations are accompanied by an increased risk of falls [19].

Dispnoea, muscle mass loss (especially in the thighs) and decreased exercise endurance will reduce the ability of COPD patients to perform daily activities and limit their exercise tolerance, creating a downward spiral that will lead to generalized immobility [20].

Difficulties in achieving day-to-day activities and related instrumental activities contribute to a reduced quality of life, but in the event of falls, devastating effects may arise on global function and even on life expectancy. Except for a major physical trauma event, the disorder is resulting in loss of functional independence and social interaction.

Several studies have shown that the history of falls in the previous year is predictive of relapse [21].

Repeated falls will lead to insecurity, fear and lack of confidence in performing daily domestic activities. In a recent study, that included 93 patients with COPD, 32% had a degree of body balance impairment during the performance of dynamic activities, compared to 5% in the control group ($p = .0005$) [22].

Fear and lack of confidence in performing everyday domestic activities will develop a chronic status of loss of movement autonomy which can lead to muscle deconditioning, higher global fatigue and greater loss of body balance. As a consequence, the adherence to treatment will decrease, especially to rehabilitation programs [19].

The most common used tests are: the Berg Balance Scale (BBS), Falls Efficacy Scale-International (FES-I), Timed Up and Go (TUG), single-leg stance test (SLS) and activities balance confidence (ABC).

Studies that tried to ascertain whether there is a correlation between COPD phenotypes and nutritional status have generated contradictory results. Some of them have found that the cachectic/emphysematous phenotype would be more prone to falls, considering that loss of skeletal muscle and weakness would be the main cause [23]. Others, by contrast, mention that the bronchitis/obese phenotype would have a higher risk of falls, due to the fact that the obese patients would record the intensity of fear more than the cachectic phenotype [24].

The overall conclusion is that patients with COPD have greater balance impairment than their healthy peers.

2.2. COPD: fundamental pathophysiological mechanisms susceptible to alter cerebral function

Cognitive impairment is multifactorial, but a history of cigarette smoking, aging and educational level are recognized as major determinants [25, 26]. The origin of the cerebral dysfunction in patients with COPD is still unknown, assuming the interference of several pathological relays: hypoxemia, oxidative stress, systemic inflammation, smoking, comorbidities, vascular-mediated brain pathology, neurotransmitter metabolism in the central nervous system (CNS), a decrease in physical functioning, genetic and epigenetic factors.

Hypoxia. In 1919, Haldane had a deep insight: "partial anoxia means not an appreciable slowing of life, but progressive, and perhaps irreparable damage to human structure." This "irreparable damage to human structure" can also include brain damage [27]. After half a century, Krop and colleagues observed the neuropsychological benefits of continuous oxygen therapy in COPD [28]. However, the first major randomized clinical trial (Nocturnal Oxygen Therapy Trials – NOTT), appeared in 1980, when the effects of continuous or nocturnal oxygen therapy on hypoxemic in COPD were investigated [29]. After the re-examination of the NOTT, it was possible to see that 42% of patients with COPD had moderate-to-severe cognitive impairment compared to 14% among controls [30]. In a follow-up of the NOTT cohort, it was observed that the neuropsychological deficit parallels the degree of hypoxia: 27% of those with mild hypoxemia to 62% in those with severe hypoxemia [31].

It is worthwhile discussing the mechanisms of response of the brain to hypoxemia. There is a very interesting mechanism for counteracting cerebral hypoxemia, the so-called cerebrovascular oxygen reactivity, which ensures blood flow up to 200% in the conditions of oxygen desaturation produced by chronic hypoxemia, nocturnal or exercise induced. For this reason, cerebral blood flow is much higher in hypoxemic than in non-hypoxemic COPD patients and even healthy controls [32, 33]. The same mechanism also explains that during rapid eye movement (REM) sleep, which accounts for about 13% of total sleep time in COPD patients, there is no cerebral hypoxemia. Surprisingly, during nonrapid eye movement (NREM) sleep, it is not known why, cerebrovascular oxygen reactivity is missing [34].

Nocturnal desaturation events are commonly met in 38–70% non-hypoxemic COPD patients [35]. Under these conditions, when the cerebrovascular oxygen reactivity mechanism is inoperative, the effect of night-time desaturation should injure the central nervous system (CNS). This was also the goal of a study of 115 non-hypoxemic COPD patients grades 2 and 3, without sleep apnoea, to which it was dosed a serum surrogate marker, namely S100B (a calcium binding protein produced in brain damage), and at the same time neuromuscular function via motor cortex activation and excitability and maximal voluntary quadriceps strength measurement was assessed. Absence of cerebrovascular reactivity would be the mechanism leading to brain injury formation during NREM sleep desaturations, which was found in approximately 50% of non-hypoxemic COPD patients [36].

The effort in daily activities would be likely to cause brain damage in severe COPD hypoxemic patients; emphasizing desaturations, inducing increase of frontal lobes choline (which is a reliable marker of myelin destruction with alteration of neuronal membrane turnover) corresponding to white matter hyperintensities on magnetic resonance imaging (MRI) [7].

In a study that enrolled younger patients (45–65 years) with COPD, low baseline oxygen saturation (≤88%) was strongly related to cognitive impairment (adjusted OR = 5.45). But what is more relevant is that in the same study, regular use of supplemental oxygen therapy in home setting decreased the risk for cognitive impairment (OR = 0.14; $P < 0.0001$) [37]. It is a recognized fact that long-term oxygen therapy (LTOT) is able to protect significantly ($p < 0.022$) the cognitive functions from COPD-induced deterioration. Another fact is that the patients with mild cognitive impairment COPD induced are unaware of the risk that involves repetitive desaturations to produce conversion from mild cognitive impairment to dementia, if nothing is done with LTOT [38, 39].

Therefore, continuous or even intermittent hypoxia (efforts, daily activities and sleep) may cause changes in brain perfusion, transient deficits in neurotransmitter metabolism in the central nervous system with changes in brain neurochemistry and structure [7, 36, 40–42].

Although hypoxia is *per se* a damaging factor, it mostly acts in an additive manner in the development of structural abnormalities in the brain [43].

Chronic systemic inflammation. Inflammation as a driving force to the central pathology of the disease, in very recent years has been subjected to doubts and contestations [44]. Even in the definition of COPD, GOLD 2017 no longer mentions the contribution of chronic inflammation to the pathophysiological process [1].

However, patients with COPD, particularly when the disease is severe and during exacerbations have evidence of systemic inflammation: increased circulating cytokine, chemokine, and acute-phase protein levels or abnormalities in circulating cells. These mediators are derived from inflammatory and structural cells in the lung and interact with each other in a complex manner. Similar mediators that are found in the lungs of patients with COPD might also be increased in the circulation, presumed reached here through translocation or "spill-over"; this chronic low-grade systemic inflammation could underlie and potentiate comorbidities (muscle wasting/cachexia, cardiovascular diseases, osteoporosis, etc.) including central nervous system impairment [45, 46]. The chronic inflammatory status may contribute to vessel wall changes (endothelial dysfunction, stiffening of arteries and arterioles and impaired vascular reactivity) and may also have neurotoxic effects: synaptic dysfunction and neural cell apoptosis [46–49].

The inflammed endothelium overexpresses surface adhesion molecules, such as vascular cell adhesion molecule-1 (VCAM-1), facilitating the adherence of white blood cells to damaged endothelial surfaces. Interleukin 6 (IL-6) can stimulate the release of acute-phase proteins by hepatocytes, including C-reactive protein (CRP), serum amyloid A, fibrinogen and procoagulant factors, which further promote or amplify the inflammatory process [50]. Moreover, CRP fosters the uptake of low-density lipoproteins (LDL) by macrophages, which contribute to the increased prevalence of arterial plaques containing a lipid core in patients with COPD [51]. Accelerated atherogenesis and impaired endothelial function, caused by a vascular inflammation status is assumed to lead to microvascular dysfunction and cerebral small vessel disease (microbleeds and lacunar infarcts) having as a consequence cognitive and functional impairment [52].

On the other hand, COPD is frequently associated with cardiovascular diseases, obesity or metabolic syndrome, the contribution of comorbidities into the systemic elevation of IL-6 levels is difficult to disentangle. Some authors described an inflammatory-prone COPD phenotype, patients with an increased risk of exacerbations (OR = 3.7) and simultaneously more severe cardiovascular and cerebral abnormalities [53, 54].

Acute exacerbations of COPD. These patients had significantly poorer cognitive function compared with control participants 3 months after discharge from hospital [55]. During a severe exacerbation, in the context of hypoxemia, paroxysmal inflammation (increased platelet activity and coagulation) and a pre-existing endothelial dysfunction, plaque rupture can occur and consequences will be coronary obstruction and stroke. However, other studies have shown that cognitive impairment during the exacerbation period recovers during periods of stability [56].

Smoking. Smoking has pleiotropic disastrous effects: promotes atherosclerosis (endothelial changes), direct effect of neurotoxicity (heavy metal, nicotine and constituents of smoke), exacerbates hypoxia brain due to chronically elevated carbon monoxide causing a left shift of the oxyhaemoglobin dissociation curve, deteriorates lung function, favors the development of comorbidities which have a negative effect on cognitive processes. Chronic smoking is also involved in the production of pathogenic changes (decrease in the gray matter density) in areas where Alzheimer's disease develops (inferior parietal lobule and precuneus). Moreover, its deleterious action can continue even after smoking cessation [57–59].

Comorbidities. It is a recognized fact that general morbidity and the burden of disease increases with both age and cumulative pathology, and COPD is no exception.

In a study of 52 stable non-hypoxic COPD patients, Ersel Dag et al., found that subjects with better functional capacity and lower comorbidity had better cognitive function; according to this study, the MoCA would be superior to Mini Mental Status Examination (MMSE) in detecting cognitive decline [60]. A higher Charlson Comorbidity Index and a reduced functional level have induced cognitive decline; this is also the conclusion of another similar study with 1 year follow-up of patients with COPD, which at baseline hospitalization lacked cognitive impairment [61]. Cleutjens et al. in a cross-sectional observational study on 90 stable COPD patients compared to 90 matched non-COPD controls, analyzed general cognitive impairment and domain-specific cognitive impairment using a complex battery of 6 psychometric tests, after correction for comorbidities using multivariate linear and logistic regression models. They found a prevalence rate of 56.7% for general cognitive impairment, which meant four times higher compared to matched non-COPD controls. The most prevalent affected domains were planning and cognitive flexibility, where abnormal planning was observed in 16.7% of patients without comorbidities but in none of the controls without comorbidities, and abnormal cognitive flexibility was observed in 44.4 and 11.6% of patients and controls without comorbidities, respectively [9].

Diseases accompanied by hypoxemia and vascular damage (coronary heart disease, cardiac failure, hypertension and stroke) have a proven risk of developing neural damage that is amplified if active smoking is also associated [4].

Another comorbidity present in over 20% of COPD cases is Obstructive Sleep Apnoea Syndrome (OSAS), a disease that underlies many common pathological pathways. Through recurrent hypoxia, moderate–severe forms of OSAS are able to affect cognitive performance, especially by focusing on attention, complex thinking, learning and memory [62, 63].

Depression and anxiety are among the most common comorbidities of COPD, reaching over 70% in oxygen-dependent cases, and much more important is that onset of depression was predictive of cognitive decline among COPD patients [64].

COPD was associated with baseline and incident disability which progresses over time and cognitive impairment was found to have an additive effect on this disability [64–66].

Therefore, cognitive comorbidities may contribute to a substantial burden of COPD-related morbidity, especially by impairing quality of life, reducing physical activity, reducing adherence to treatment and increasing the frequency of hospital admission.

Oxidative stress. An increase in the level of reactive oxygen species (oxygen ions, free radicals and peroxides) leads to oxidative stress, which would alter the neuronal signals that produce neuro-inflammation with neuro-degeneration and implicitly with cognitive impairment [67]. The most important triggers for the development of oxidative stress in patients with COPD are cigarette smoke and systemic inflammation.

Other possible mechanisms. In a highly laborious study in 55 patients with moderate-severe COPD in stable period were determined: (i) cognitive ability (through a battery of 6 psychometric tests), (ii) structural brain abnormalities using 3T MRI to seek signs of small vessels disease (white matter hyperintensities, lacunes, cerebral microbleeds and enlarged perivascular spaces) and (iii) hippocampal volume as an area involved in memory process. The 55 patients were divided into 2 subgroups, cognitively high (25 patients) and low-performing (30 patients), having comparable demographics, clinical characteristics and comorbidities. No structural changes were found between COPD patients with low or high cognitive performance, demonstrating that small vessels disease would not represent a pathological pathway [68]. On the contrary, other authors provided evidence of significant white and gray matter abnormalities associated with cognitive dysfunction in patients with COPD without arterial hypoxemia or hypercapnia. Given the paucity in current evidence, more research is needed to evaluate the impact of cerebral small vessel disease on stroke and cognitive functioning in patients with COPD [69, 70].

Mitochondria are the intracellular organelles that provide aerobic respiration and cellular energy. As a result, mitochondrial diseases have as expression and localization the most oxygen-consuming tissues: skeletal muscles, central nervous system and heart. Depending on the load of mutant mitochondrial genomes, neurological expression ranges from mild cognitive impairment to dementia, or epilepsy, stroke-like episodes, ataxia, etc. In COPD, there are approximately 20% of cachexia cases in which a mitochondrial component might be involved [71, 72].

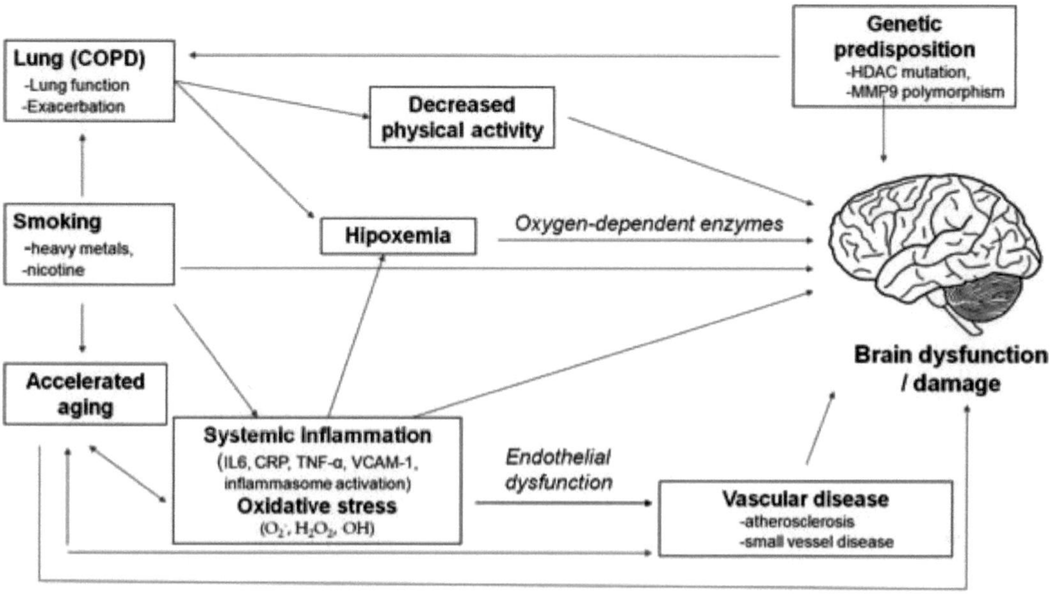

Figure 1. Potential mechanisms contributing to brain dysfunction and/or damage in elderly subjects with COPD. HDAC: histone deacetylase, MMP9: matrix metalloproteinase 9, IL-6: interleukin 6, CRP: C-reactive protein, TNF-α: tumor necrosis factor, VCAM-1: vascular cell adhesion molecule-1.

Many factors, generated by, or interconnected with COPD, could contribute to brain dysfunction and/or damage (**Figure 1**).

2.3. Clinical consequences of an affected cognition; measure methods

In order to diagnose MCI, besides the clinical and anamnestic examination, psychometric tests as well as neurochemistry and neuroimaging assessment are available.

Torres-Sánchez et al., in their meta-analysis listed more than 40 psychometric tests that were used [73]. The most used psychometric questionnaires are: the Mini Mental Status Examination (MMSE), the Clock Drawing test, the Trail Making test (TMT) A, the TMT B, Memory Impairment Screen (MIS); Montreal Cognitive Assessment test (MoCA) [74]. It is advisable to use a battery of tests, not a single one, to improve the result accuracy [75, 76].

Neuroimaging studies showed there are significantly lowered gray matter volumes in several brain regions as hippocamp [7], limbic and paralimbic structures [77], precuneus, bilateral calcarine, right superior temporal gyrus/middle temporal gyrus, bilateral fusiform, right inferior parietal lobule [78], cingulate and amygdala [8], dorsolateral prefrontal cortex [77] etc., evidenced by different neuroimaging techniques based on magnetic resonance imaging (MRI). Performance accuracy has increased by introducing voxel-based morphometry analysis also based on MRI. Using this technique, it was possible to show for the first time gray matter volume alterations in stable COPD patients, even to those with subclinical cognitive impairment [79].

Passing over the slight contradictions or discrepancies between the results offered by these and other neuroimaging studies, what is common is heterogeneity and broad distribution of the lesions. Another important finding of neuroimaging studies is inferior parietal lobule and precuneus that are two regions altered also in COPD and Alzheimer disease.

Chronic airway involvement can be perceived as a strong aging factor leading to an early deterioration of cognition with a 10–15 years advanced age [2]. In a study on 301 stable moderate-severe COPD patients conducted by Schure et al. showed that cognitive functioning (especially, psychomotor speed and executive control) present in approximately 30% of cases would be associated with greater disease severity and poorer physical functioning (as measured by the six-minute walk test, total steps per day and grip strength). And these results are more relevant as patients were "healthier" COPD, namely the patients without comorbidities known underlying inflammation (Charlson Index = 0.9–1.2) [80].

Due to the non-homogeneous distribution on the brain mapping, patients will experience various and multiple disorders, most of which are reflected by difficulties in naming, memory, visuospatial, executive function and mood decrements.

COPD-related dyspnoea is a strong driver to anxiety, panic or/and depression and reduced quality of life. But, development of a secondary cognitive impairment component may contribute to increased behavioral disturbances; these may distress much more the family caregivers which need to cope with behavioral changes.

In a study on 88 patients with COPD, Turan et al. showed a positive correlation between declining of cognitive function, assessed by MMSE questionnaire, and suboptimal inhalation adherence, increasing hospitalizations and emergency visits [81]. In another study of 265 patients with COPD, adherence was measured using a tool incorporating sophisticated electronic devices to mark time and correctness of the technique; adherence over the study was 22.9% of what would be expected if all the doses had been taken correctly and on time, but more important adherence was negatively influenced by impairment in cognitive function [82].

According to statistics, 41% of patients with stable COPD who undergo rehabilitation would suffer from any cognitive impairment. Inclusion and completion of a pulmonary rehabilitation program is however affected by the presence of cognitive impairment, the drop-out number being higher in those with cognitive impairment. However, the comparison of the different parameters (functional status, health status and psychological well-being) to the patients able to complete the program does not differ between cognitive impairment patients and those with no cognitive impairment, this being an argument that patients suffering from cognitive impairment can benefit from the programs rehabilitation [83]. Do not forget to investigate factors related to balance changes in patients with COPD. Although the risk of falls may seem less important than the consequences of COPD itself, falls are associated with increased mortality, reduced independence, poorer quality of life and lower level of physical activity.

Depression and anxiety are found in high proportions (30–70%) and identifying the coping styles in patients with COPD represent an important aspect of the individualized treatment of the patient, because the coping style can be both adaptive, implying the stress reduction and maladaptive, situation in which the maintenance and the amplification of the current symptomatology are present or can determine the appearance of some new symptomatic elements and behaviors [84].

The fact that cognitive impairment would occur at younger age [2], would cross a subclinical period [79] and would present at least 30% of cases [80], all of which signals us that cognitive impairment may be an early indicator of emerging risk of frailty and poor overall mental functioning among COPD patients.

Cognitive impairment has also been reported to worsen over time due to both the aggravation of COPD and the increase in burden represented by the progression and/or complications of comorbidities [85]. Chang et al. reported that the co-occurrence of COPD and cognitive impairment in a 3-year prospective study was associated with increased rate of disability, hospital admission and mortality [86].

3. Therapeutic implications; preventive strategies

How to deal with a COPD patient who might be suffering from cognitive impairment? Based on growing evidence in recent years, it is reasonable that cognitive assessment in subjects suffering from chronic obstructive disease should enter the routine of diagnostic procedures to grade the overall impact of patients' respiratory condition. Multiple areas of cognition being altered in varying degrees, may explain a poor awareness of the disease and may compromise the individual's ability to manage his or her own care and adherence to treatment. The clinician, who observes signs of forgetfulness, disorientation or balance trouble and/or even poor adherence to medical treatment, should prompt to conduct further assessments using screening tools (e.g. MMSE score).

Addressing comorbidities. The number of comorbidities increases with age progression. Specific attention must be focused on so-called cognitive comorbidities. They relate in particular to cardiovascular diseases, cerebrovascular diseases, diabetes mellitus and OSAS. These should be treated according to current guidelines.

Pulmonary rehabilitation. Balance training and fall prevention strategies are not included in international guidelines for PR, and very few programs include standardized balance assessment. Although exercise can improve balance and decrease fall risk in older adults, interventions that include exercise to challenge balance have greater effects on fall risk and balance. Physical exercise training involving balance, strength training, movement speed and coordination has improved balance and frailty markers in multiple randomized and nonrandomized studies [87, 88]. Past cross-sectional research has provided support for the hypothesis that greater levels of aerobic fitness may be associated with a lessening of the normal age-related declines in cognitive functioning [89, 90]. It is conceivable that improvements in cognitive functions such as executive function might help to improve self-management skills and potentially assist in sustaining the other substantial benefits of pulmonary rehabilitation.

Cognitive training. Given the increased prevalence of cognitive impairment in COPD and potentially devastating effects, a structured assessment of cognitive function should be implemented as a routine component of the evaluation of COPD patients. Those identified with a screening tool as possibly having MCI should be referred for further assessment to a psychiatrist. Identifying the coping styles in patients with COPD represents an important aspect of the individualized treatment of the patient. Interventions aiming at enhancing the problem- or emotion-focused coping may improve COPD prognosis [91].

Oxygen therapy: to whom? when? There is debate whether screening for cognitive impairment should be routinely applied. From the point of view of the hypoxemia approach, the answer to this debate will have to consider the evidence: (1) one in four people with COPD have cognitive impairment and over time, cognitive decline will deepen (risking an evolution toward multi-infarct dementia or Alzheimer disease) [92–94]. (2) It is now recognized that not only continuous, but also intermittent hypoxia (efforts, daily activities and sleep) can by repetition cause changes in brain neurochemistry and structure [7, 36]. (3) Cognitive impairment goes along with the severity of COPD, age and type/number of cognitive comorbidities. (4) Regular use of supplemental oxygen therapy has been shown to decrease the risk for cognitive impairment in patients with COPD [37, 38, 95].

Therefore, even the detection of intermittent desaturation (effort, daily activity and sleep), will have to lead to establishing earlier oxygen supplementation in order to prevent irreversible brain damage.

4. Conclusions

At least 40% of COPD patients present irreversible neuronal damage or dysfunction that is separate from other comorbidities. That is why cognitive impairment has to be listed in the first line of extrathoracic manifestations. Not identifying cognitive impairment we miss the fact that this condition may be a precursor to develop dementia in about a third of cases, or even higher in the context of COPD associated with other comorbidities. Cognitive impairment has been shown to increase the risk of hospitalization, disability and death. Hypoxemia is a serious problem that, even under the conditions of intermittent occurrence, should be sanctioned as early as possible by establishing LTOT. Besides oxygen therapy, the most effective therapeutic actions and strategies to these particular populations include: addressing comorbidities, pulmonary rehabilitation and cognitive training.

Author details

Cristian Oancea*, Emanuela Tudorache and Voicu Tudorache

*Address all correspondence to: oancea@umft.ro

Department of Pulmonology, University of Medicine and Pharmacy, Timisoara, Romania

References

[1] Global Initiative for Chronic Obstructive Lung Disease, 2017. http://goldcopd.org/wp-content/uploads/2016/12/wms-GOLD-2017-Pocket-Guide.pdf page.2

[2] Roberto W, Negro D, Bonadiman L, Tognella S, et al. Extent and prevalence of cognitive dysfunction in chronic obstructive pulmonary disease, chronic non-obstructive bronchitis, and in asymptomatic smokers, compared to normal reference values. International Journal of COPD. 2014;**9**:675-683

[3] Petersen RC, Smith GE, Waring SC, et al. Mild cognitive impairment: Clinical characterization and outcome. Archives of Neurology. 1999;**56**:303-308

[4] Yohannes AM, Chen W, Moga AM, et al. Cognitive impairment in chronic obstructive pulmonary disease and chronic heart failure: A systematic review and meta-analysis of observational studies. JAMDA. May 1;**18**(5):451.e1-451.e11

[5] Langa KM, Levine DA. The diagnosis and management of mild cognitive impairment. A clinical review. JAMA. 2014;**32**:2551-2561

[6] Dodd JW, Getov SV, Jones PW. Cognitive function in COPD. The European Respiratory Journal. 2010;**35**:913-922

[7] Borson S, Scanlan J, Friedman S, et al. Modeling the impact of COPD on the brain. International Journal of COPD. 2008;**3**(3):429-434

[8] Roland W, Esser M, Stoeckel C, Kirsten A, et al. Structural brain changes in patients with COPD. Chest. 2016;**149**(2):426-434

[9] Cleutjens FAHM, Franssen FME, Spruit MA, et al. Domain-specific cognitive impairment in patients with COPD and control subjects. International Journal of COPD. 2017;**12**:1-11

[10] Kuo HK, Jones RN, Milberg WP, et al. Effect of blood pressure and diabetes mellitus on cognitive and physical functions in older adults: A longitudinal analysis of the advanced cognitive training for independent and vital elderly cohort. Journal of the American Geriatrics Society. 2005;**53**:1154-1161

[11] López-Torres I, Valenza MC, Torres-Sánchez I, et al. Changes in cognitive status in COPD patients across clinical stages. COPD: Journal of Chronic Obstructive Pulmonary Disease. Dec 2015;14 Jun;**13**(3):327-32. DOI: 10.3109/15412555.2015.1081883

[12] Thakur N, Blanc PD, Julian LJ, et al. COPD and cognitive impairment: The role of hypoxemia and oxygen therapy. International Journal of Chronic Obstructive Pulmonary Disease. 2010;**5**:263-269

[13] Grant I, Heaton RK, McSweeny AJ, Adams KM, Timms RM. Neuropsychologic findings in hypoxemic chronic obstructive pulmonary disease. Archives of Internal Medicine. 1982;**142**(8):1470-1476

[14] Tudorache E, Oancea C, Avram C, et al. Balance impairment and systemic inflammation in chronic obstructive pulmonary disease. International Journal of COPD. 2015;**10**:1847-1852

[15] Rubenstein LZ. Falls in older people: Epidemiology, risk factors and strategies for prevention. Age and Ageing. 2006;**35**:37-41

[16] Roig M, Eng JJ, MacIntyre DL, et al. Falls in people with chronic obstructive pulmonary disease: An observational cohort study. Respiratory Medicine. 2011;**105**(3):461-469

[17] Roig M, Eng JJ, MacIntyre DL, Road JD. Falls in patients with chronic obstructive pulmonary disease: A call for further research. Respiratory Medicine. 2009;**103**(9):1257-1269

[18] Agusti A, Calverley PM, Celli B, et al., Evaluation of COPD longitudinally to identify predictive surrogate endpoints (ECLIPSE) investigators. Characterisation of COPD heterogeneity in the ECLIPSE cohort. Respiratory Research. 2010, Sep 10;**11**:122. DOI: 10.1186/1465-9921-11-122

[19] Crişan AF, Oancea C, Timar B, Fira-Mladinescu O, Tudorache V. Balance impairment in patients with COPD. PloS One. 2015 March; 13;**10**(3):e0120573

[20] Wouters EF. Chronic obstructive pulmonary disease. 5: Systemic effects of COPD. Thorax. 2002;**57**:1067-1070

[21] Beauchamp MK, Hill K, Goldstein RS, et al. Impairments in balance discriminate fallers from non-fallers in COPD. Chest. 2012;**141**(6):1496-1503

[22] Porto EF, Pradella CO, Rocco CM, et al. Comparative postural control in COPD patients and healthy individuals during dynamic and static activities. Journal of Cardiopulmonary Rehabilitation and Prevention. 2017;**37**:139-145

[23] Ko S, Stenholm S, Ferrucci L. Characteristic gait patterns in older adults with obesity – Results from the Baltimore longitudinal study of aging. Journal of Biomechanics. 2010;**43**:1104-1110

[24] Voica AS, Oancea C, Tudorache E, et al. Chronic obstructive pulmonary disease phenotypes and balance impairment. International Journal of COPD. 2016;**11**:919-925

[25] Barnes JN. Exercise, cognitive function, and aging. Advances in Physiology Education. 2015;**39**(2):55-62

[26] Roncero C, Campuzano AI, Quintano JA, et al. Cognitive status among patients with chronic obstructive pulmonary disease. International Journal of COPD. 2016;**11**:543-551

[27] Haldane JS. Symptoms, causes, and prevention of anoxemia (Insufficient Supply of Oxygen to the Tissues), and the value of oxygen in its treatment. British Medical Journal. Jul 19;**2**(3055):65-72

[28] Krop HD, Block AJ, Cohen E. Neuropsychologic effects of continuous oxygen therapy in chronic obstructive pulmonary disease. Chest. 1973;**64**:317-322

[29] Continuous or nocturnal oxygen therapy in hypoxemic chronic obstructive lung disease: a clinical trial. Nocturnal Oxygen Therapy Trial Group. Annals of Internal Medicine. 1980;**93**:391-398

[30] Heaton RK, Grant I, McSweeny AJ, et al. Psychologic effects of continuous and nocturnal oxygen therapy in hypoxemic chronic obstructive pulmonary disease. Archives of Internal Medicine. 1983;**143**(10):1941-1947

[31] Grant I, Prigatano GP, Heaton RK, et al. Progressive neuropsychologic impairment and hypoxemia. Relationship in chronic obstructive pulmonary disease. Archives of General Psychiatry. 1987;**44**:999-1006

[32] Albayrak R, Fidan F, Unlu M, et al. Extracranial carotid Dopplerultrasound evaluation of cerebral blood flow volume in COPD patients. Respiratory Medicine. 2006;**100**:1826-1833

[33] Yildiz S, Kaya I, Cece H, et al. Impact of COPD exacerbation on cerebral blood flow. Clinical Imaging. 2012;**36**:185-190

[34] Meadows GE, O'Driscoll DM, Simonds AK, et al. Cerebral blood flow response to isocapnic hypoxia during slow-wave sleep and wakefulness. Journal of Applied Physiology. 2004;**97**:1343-1348

[35] Lacasse Y, Series F, Vujovic-Zotovic N, et al. Evaluating nocturnal oxygen desaturation in COPD--revised. Respiratory Medicine. 2011;**105**:1331-1337

[36] Alexandre F, Heraud N, Sanchez AMJ, et al. Brain damage and motor cortex impairment in chronic obstructive pulmonary disease: Implication of nonrapid eye movement SLEEP desaturation. Sleep. 2016;**39**(2):327-35

[37] Thakur N, Blanc PD, Julian LJ, et al. COPD and cognitive impairment: The role of hypoxemia and oxygen therapy. International Journal of Chronic Obstructive Pulmonary Disease. 2010;**5**:263-269

[38] Karamanli H, Ilik F, Kayhan F, et al. Assessment of cognitive impairment in long-term oxygen therapy-dependent COPD patients. International Journal of COPD. 2015;**10**:2087-2094

[39] Dal Negro RW, Bonadiman L, Bricolo FP, Tognella S, Turco P. Cognitive dysfunction in severe chronic obstructive pulmonary disease (COPD) with or without long-term oxygen therapy (LTOT). Multidisciplinary Respiratory Medicine. 2015 Apr 19;**10**(1):17

[40] Ortapamuk H, Naldoken S. Brain perfusion abnormalities in chronic obstructive pulmonary disease: Comparison with cognitive impairment. Annals of Nuclear Medicine. 2006;**20**(2):99-106

[41] Gibson GE, Pulsinelli W, Blass JP, Duffy TE. Brain dysfunction in mild to moderate hypoxia. The American Journal of Medicine. 1981;**70**(6):1247-1254

[42] Maccioni RB, Rojo LE, Fernandez JA, Kuljis RO. The role of neuroimmunomodulation in Alzheimer's disease. Annals of the New York Academy of Sciences. 2009;**1153**:240-246

[43] Huppert FA. Memory impairment associated with chronic hypoxia. Thorax. 1982;**37**(11): 858-860

[44] Eapen MS, Myers S, Walters EH, et al. Airway inflammation in chronic obstructive pulmonary diseases: a true paradox. Expert Review of Respiratory Medicine. DOI: 10.1080/17476348.2017.1360769

[45] Barnes PJ, Celli BR. Systemic manifestations and comorbidities of COPD. The European Respiratory Journal. 2009;**33**:1165-1185

[46] Barnes PJ. Mechanisms of allergic diseases. The Journal of Allergy and Clinical Immunology. 2016;**138**:16-27

[47] Gan WQ, Man SF, Senthilselvan A, Sin DD. Association between chronic obstructive pulmonary disease and systemic inflammation: A systematic review and a meta-analysis. Thorax. 2004;**59**(7):574-580

[48] Su B, Liu T, Fan H, et al. Inflammatory markers and the risk of chronic obstructive pulmonary disease: A systematic review and meta-analysis. PloS One. 2016;**11**:e0150586

[49] Gorska-Ciebiada M, Saryusz-Wolska M, Borkowska A, et al. Serum levels of inflammatory markers in depressed elderly patients with diabetes and mild cognitive impairment. PloS One. 2015;**10**:e0120433

[50] Sin DD, Anthonisen NR, Soriano JB, Agusti AG. Mortality in COPD: Role ofncomorbidities. The European Respiratory Journal. 2006;**28**(6):1245-1257

[51] Sin DD, MacNee W. Chronic obstructive pulmonary disease and cardiovascular diseases: A "vulnerable" relationship. American Journal of Respiratory and Critical Care Medicine. 2013;**187**(1):2-4

[52] Lahousse L, Q. van den Bouwhuijsen, D.W. Loth, et al., Chronic obstructive pulmonary disease and lipid core carotid artery plaques in the elderly: The rotterdam study, American Journal of Respiratory and Critical Care Medicine. 2013;**187**(1):58-64

[53] Agusti A et al. Persistent systemic inflammation is associated with poor clinical outcomes in COPD: A novel phenotype. PloS One. 2012;**7**(5):e37483

[54] Thomson M, Ingebrigtsen TS, Marrot JL, et al. Inflammatory biomarkers and exacerbations in COPD. JAMA. June, 12, 2013;**309**(22):2353-61

[55] Dodd JW, Charlton RA, van den Broek MD, Jones PW. Cognitive dysfunction in patients hospitalized with acute exacerbation of COPD. Chest 2013;**144**(1):119-127

[56] Ambrosino N, Bruletti G, Scala V, et al. Cognitive and perceived health status in patient with chronic obstructive pulmonary disease surviving acute on chronic respiratory failure: A controlled study. Intensive Care Medicine. 2002;**28**(2):170-177

[57] Krueger CE, Dean DL, Rosen HJ, et al. Longitudinal rates of lobar atrophy in frontotemporal dementia, semantic dementia, and Alzheimer's disease. Alzheimer Disease and Associated Disorders. 2010;**24**:43-48

[58] Jan Ankersmit H, Nickl S, Hoeltl E, et al. Increased serum levels of HSP27 as a marker for incipient chronic obstructive pulmonary disease in young smokers. Respiration. 2012;**83**:391-399

[59] Lahousse L, Tiemeier H, Ikram MA, Brusselle GG. Chronic obstructive pulmonary disease and cerebrovascular disease: A comprehensive review. Respiratory Medicine. 2015;**109**:1371-1380

[60] Dag E, Bulcun E, Turkel Y, et al. Factors influencing cognitive function in subjects with COPD. Respiratory Care. 01, March 2016; DOI: 10.4187/respcare.04403

[61] Helvik AS, Selbæk G, Engedal K. Cognitive decline one year after hospitalization in older adults without dementia. Dementia and Geriatric Cognitive Disorders. 2012;**34**(3):198-205

[62] Fletcher EC. Chronic lung disease in the sleep apnea syndrome. Lung. 1990;**168**:751-761

[63] Engleman HM, Douglas NJ. Sleep 4: Sleepiness, cognitive function, and quality of life in obstructive sleep apnoea/hypopnoea syndrome. Thorax. 2004;**59**:618-662

[64] Incalzi RA, Chiappini F. Fuso, et al., predicting cognitive decline in patients with hypoxaemic COPD. Respiratory Medicine. 1998;**92**(3):527-533

[65] Martinez C, Richardson C, Han M, Cigolle C, et al. Chronic obstructive pulmonary disease, cognitive impairment, and development of disability: The health and retirement study. Annals of the American Thoracic Society. 2014;**11**:1362-1370

[66] Pedone C et al. Drawing impairment predicts mortality in severe COPD. Chest. 2006; **130**(6):1687-1694

[67] Popa-Wagner A, Mitran S, Sivanesan S, et al. ROS and brain diseases: The good, the bad, and the ugly. Oxidative Medicine and Cellular Longevity. 2013;**963520**. DOI: 10.1155/2013/963520

[68] Cleutjens FAHM, Ponds RWHM, Spruit MA, et al. The Relationship between Cerebral Small Vessel Disease, Hippocampal Volume and Cognitive Functioning in Patients with COPD: An MRI Study. Frontiers in Aging Neuroscience. 1 March 2017;**9**(88):1-9. DOI: 10.3389/fnagi.2017.00088

[69] Pantoni L. Cerebral small vessel disease: From pathogenesis and clinical characteristics to therapeutic challenges. Lancet Neurology. 2010;**9**(7):689-701

[70] Cai Z, Wang C, He W, Tu H, Tang Z, Xiao M, et al. Cerebral small vessel disease and Alzheimer's disease. Clinical Interventions in Aging. 2015;**10**:1695-1704

[71] Mancuso M, Calsolaro V, Orsucci D, et al. Mitochondria, cognitive impairment, and Alzheimer's disease. International Journal of Alzheimer's Disease. 2009;**2009**(951548). DOI: 10.4061/2009/951548

[72] Cielen N, Maes K, Gayan-Ramirez G. Musculoskeletal disorders in chronic obstructive pulmonary disease. BioMed Research International. 2014;**2014**(965764):1-17. DOI: 10.1155/2014/965764

[73] Torres-Sánchez I, Rodríguez-Alzueta E, Cabrera-Martos I, et al. Cognitive impairment in COPD: A systematic review. Jornal Brasileiro de Pneumologia. 2015;**41**(2):182-190

[74] Crisan AF, Oancea C, Timar B, Fira-Mladinescu O, Crisan A, Tudorache V. Cognitive Impairment in Chronic Obstructive Pulmonary Disease. PloS One. July 2014;**9**(7): e102468. DOI: 10.1371/journal.pone.0102468

[75] Trzepacz PT, Hochstetler H, Wang S, et al. Alzheimer's Disease Neuroimaging Initiative. Relationship between the Montreal cognitive assessment and Mini mental state examination for assessment of mild cognitive impairment in older adults. BMC Geriatrics. 2015;**15**:107

[76] Cameron J, Worrall-Carter L, Page K, et al. Screening for mild cognitive impairment in patients with heart failure: Montreal Cognitive Assessment versus Mini Mental State Exam. European Journal of Cardiovascular Nursing. 2013;**12**:252-260

[77] Zhang H, Wang X, Lin J, et al. Reduced regional gray matter volume in patients with chronic obstructive pulmonary disease: A voxel-based morphometry study. American Journal of Neuroradiology. 2013;**34**:334-339

[78] Wang C, Ding Y, Shen B, et al. Altered Gray matter volume in stable chronic obstructive pulmonary disease with subclinical cognitive impairment: An exploratory study. Neurotoxicity Research, Published Online. 22 December 2016; DOI: 10.1007/s12640-016-9690-9

[79] Chen J, Lin IT, Zhang H, et al. Reduced cortical thickness, surface area in patients with chronic obstructive pulmonary disease: A surface-based morphometry and neuropsychological study. Brain Imaging and Behavior. 2016;**10**:464-476

[80] Schure MB, Borson S, Nguyen HQ, et al. Fan associations of cognition with physical functioning and health-related quality of life among COPD patients. Respiratory Medicine. 9 March, 2016;**114**:46-52. DOI: 10.1016/j.rmed.2016.03.005

[81] Turan O, Turan PA, Mirici A. Parameters affecting inhalation therapy adherence in elderly patients with chronic obstructive lung disease and asthma. Geriatrics & Gerontology International. 2016; Jun;**17**(6):999-1005. DOI: 10.1111/ggi.12823

[82] Sulaiman I, Cushen B, Greene G, et al. Objective assessment of adherence to inhalers by COPD patients. AJRCCM. Articles in Press. Published on 13-July-2016 May 15;**195**(10):1333-1343. DOI: 10.1164/rccm.201604-0733OC

[83] Cleutjens FAHM, Spruit MA, Ponds RWHM, et al. The impact of cognitive impairment on efficacy of pulmonary rehabilitation in patients with COPD. JAMDA. 2016;1-7

[84] Maes S, Leventhal H, de Ridder DTD. Coping with chronic illness. In: Zeidner M, Endler NS, editors. Handbook of Coping. New York: Wiley & Sons; May 1;**18**(5):420-426

[85] Fix AJ, Daughton D, Kass I, Bell CW, Golden CJ. Cognitive functioning and survival among patients with chronic obstructive pulmonary disease. The International Journal of Neuroscience. 1985;**27**(1-2):13-17

[86] Chang SS, Chen S, McAvay GJ, Tinetti ME. Effect of coexisting chronic obstructive pulmonary disease and cognitive impairment on health outcomes in older adults. Journal of the American Geriatrics Society. 2012;**60**:1839-1846

[87] Chin A Paw MJM, van Uffelen JGZ, Riphagen I., The functional effects of physical exercise TRaining in frail older people. A systematic review., Sports Medicine, 2008; **38**:781-793

[88] Binder EF, Schechtman KB, Ehsani AA, et al. Effects of exercise training on frailty in community-dwelling older adults: Results of a randomized, controlled trial. Journal of the American Geriatrics Society. 2002;**50**:1921-1928

[89] Clarkson-Smith L, Hartley AA. Relationships between physical exercise and cognitive abilities in older adults. Psychology and Aging. 1989;**4**:183-189

[90] Elsayed M, Ismail AH, Young RJ. Intellectual differences of adult men related to age and physical fitness before and after an exercise program. Journal of Gerontology. 1980;**35**:383-387

[91] Papava I, Oancea C, Enatescu VR, et al. The impact of coping on the somatic and mental status of patients with COPD: A cross-sectional study. International Journal of COPD. 2016;**11**:1343-1351

[92] Hung W, Wisnivesky JP, Siu AL, et al. Cognitive decline among patients with chronic obstructive pulmonary disease. American Journal of Respiratory and Critical Care Medicine. 2009;**180**(2):134-137

[93] Ma F, Wu T, Miao R, et al. Conversion of mild cognitive impairment to dementia among subjects with diabetes: A population-based study of incidence and risk factors with five years of follow-up. Journal of Alzheimer's Disease. 2015;**43**:1441-1449

[94] Gauthier S, Reisberg B, Zaudig M, et al. International psychogeriatric association expert conference on mild cognitive impairment: Mild cognitive impairment. Lancet. 2006;**367**(9518):1262-1270

[95] Long Term Oxygen Therapy (LTOT). Thomas L. Petty., Robert W. McCoy., Dennis E. Doherty, 6th Oxygen Consensus Conference Recommendations., 2006

Section 2

Updates in Smoking Cessation and Pulmonary Rehabilitation

Chapter 5

Tobacco and Smoking Cessation

Thomas Hering

Additional information is available at the end of the chapter

http://dx.doi.org/10.5772/intechopen.70565

Abstract

Smoking cessation is essential for COPD patients. It mitigates the progression of the disease and the loss of ventilatory capacity, thus improving the overall prognosis. Overall mortality can be reduced effectively including mortality from respiratory diseases as well as lung cancer and cardiovascular diseases. Its main goal must be to initiate tobacco cessation as early as possible after diagnosing COPD so as to enable the patient to influence the course of this disease in the most effective way possible. Depending on the degree of tobacco addiction, the application of behavioural therapy combined with pharmaceutical support has shown to be the most reliable therapy with highest long-term abstinence rates. Particular consideration is needed for patients with psychiatric comorbidity mainly represented by depression. The setting of tobacco cessation measures in outpatient clinics or practices embedded in long-term therapy of the underlying respiratory disease appears to be crucial for long-time abstinence.

Keywords: smoking cessation, behavioural therapy, nicotine replacement, varenicline, bupropione, abstinence rates, e-cigarette

1. Introduction

In continuous long-term smokers, the exposition of the bronchial mucosa to the toxic components of cigarette smoke results in a progressive inflammatory process with the consequence of functional and structural destruction of the airways. Thus, the ventilatory capacity in terms of respiratory volumes FEV1 and VC is reduced and hyperinflation/development of emphysema is increased in accelerated speed and patients face respiratory failure with stepwise progression of the disease [1–3]. After progression of lung function loss, gas exchange for oxygen and carbon dioxide is compromised resulting in hypoxaemia and hypercapnia. The patient's exercise ability is reduced to a minimum bringing him into the position that he needs help in even basic daily activities. Pharmaceutical therapy to relieve—mostly inhalation therapy—will not be a sufficient intervention and long-term oxygen therapy, nocturnal ventilation therapy, volume reduction measures up to lung transplantation may be considered. In addition as a consequence of the mucosa destruction, the bronchial system progressively loses the ability of mucociliary clearance resulting in higher deposition rates of the toxic components of smoke, thus enabling these substances to act carcinogenic. Consequently, continuous smokers with COPD show higher lung cancer rates compared to non-COPD individuals [4–6]. Smoking cessation, thus, must be the first measure to be taken in the treatment of COPD patients at the earliest possible time. Yet, in spite of this knowledge, a great proportion continues smoking due to various barriers among which the high degree of addiction is to be mentioned in the first place. Moreover, physicians sometimes consider smoking cessation therapy as addiction therapy as not their business or state that the majority of and former smokers had stopped on their own and by pure willpower [7], or out of section non-predictable "catastrophic" decision [8], thus neglecting the urgent need to stop the toxic smoke exposition of the bronchi as early as possible. The earlier tobacco consumption is stopped, the less the disease will develop and compromise the patient's prognosis.

2. Evidence and rationale of smoking cessation in COPD patients

Smoking is the main cause of COPD. Close to 90% of patients with COPD have a continuous smoking history. One of three continuous smokers develops COPD disease [9–12].

Susceptibility to smoke differs in gender and races. Women have a higher susceptibility to smoke compared to men, the same applies to African-American people compared to Caucasians [13–16].

Smoking and COPD represent a maximal risk for lung cancer. COPD increases the risk of developing lung cancer possibly due to the loss of the clearing capacity of the mucociliary system as a result of toxic impact of tobacco smoke. The underlying mechanisms of cellular and molecular transformation and alteration are subjects of further research, whereas the close relationship of the exceeding probability of lung cancer in COPD patients is clear [4, 17–21].

Smoking cessation allows increase of lung function in patients with COPD. A 1-year follow-up after smoking cessation shows a limited increase in lung function in COPD patients [3].

Smoking cessation allows optimal preservation of remaining ventilatory capacity in patients with COPD. Long-term observation of the course of lung function shows a lower year by year decrease after smoking cessation compared to continuous smokers who failed to stop [3, 22].

Only smoking cessation effectively leads to longer survival in COPD patients by the prevention of progression towards respiratory impairment and failure. One of the main results of the lung health study is the evidence for longer survival in COPD patients after 14.5 years [23].

Smoking cessation allows the improvement of coughing, shortness of breath and bronchitis within weeks. Within only 4 weeks, a marked decrease of coughing and bronchitis symptoms as well as shortness of breath is observed after smoking cessation [24].

http://dx.doi.org/10.5772/intechopen.70565

3. Smoking cessation: motivation, methods and techniques

Smoking cessation as the main measure for treating COPD patients who still smoke is very well established in guidelines on an international and national basis an in Cochrane Reviews [25, 26].

3.1. Motivational interviewing strategy

Motivational interviewing (MI) technique [27] is a fundamental tool for initial motivation.

Primary motivation towards tobacco cessation is essential to start patient's action. Motivational interviewing technique has showed to be most effective and time effective at this end. The technique consists, in short, in interviewing the patient himself on his own attitudes towards his smoking while respecting his autonomy. While doing so, the patient will produce his main possible reasons in favour of smoking cessation like health concerns, financial issues, aspects of beauty/concerns of premature ageing, being a good example for the children etc. While explaining these reasons to the interviewer, the patient will influence his own tendency to move towards cessation and thus increasing the level of his own motivation for action.

3.2. The 5A-strategy and the 5R-strategy

The therapists duty is to increase the patient's understanding and motivation. Clinicians can make a difference with even a minimal (less than 3 minutes) intervention. A relation exists between the intensity of intervention and tobacco cessation outcome. Even when patients are not willing to make a quit attempt at this time, clinician-delivered brief interventions enhance motivation and increase the likelihood of future quit attempts [28]. Tobacco users are being primed to consider quitting by a wide range of societal and environmental factors (e.g., public health messages, policy changes, cessation marketing messages, family members). There is an evidence that smokers who receive clinician advice and assistance with quitting report greater satisfaction with their health care than those who do not [29, 30]. The goal of these strategies is clear: to change clinical culture and practice patterns to ensure that every patient who uses tobacco is identified. Several observations are relevant to this theme. Although many smokers are reluctant to seek intensive treatments, they nevertheless can receive a brief intervention every time they visit. The time limits on physicians as well as reimbursement restrictions, often limit providers to brief interventions, although more intensive interventions would produce greater success.

The **5A technique** (see **Table 1**) includes to "ask, advise, assess, assist, arrange…" [25].

Ask: at every single encounter, the patient is asked whether he is a smoker and how much the consumption is.

Advise: smokers will be given the clear advice to stop smoking for health considerations.

Assess: the smoker's willingness to take action for smoking cessation is to be assessed.

Assist: in case of the smokers willingness to quit she/he shall be given assistance to do so.

Arrange: follow-up is to be arranged to support success.

Ask	At every single encounter, the patient is asked whether he is a smoker and how much the consumption is. Patients who are most repeatedly will expect the question in subsequent meetings. This by itself increases the ambivalence towards the individual smoking behaviour.
Advise	Smokers will be given the clear advice to stop smoking for health considerations. The advice must be clear without possible evasions as to the "if" and "when." If this advice is not been given by the physician, the patient will interpret it as active permission to continue smoking.
Assess	The smoker's willingness to take action for smoking cessation is to be assessed. If there is a substantial willingness to quit, the patient must be given a detailed possible instruction to proceed. Often, the first hint may be the patient asking for more information on how to proceed. Detailed information then shall be given in a neutral way respecting the patient's autonomy regarding his decision for the next step.
Assist	In case of the smokers willingness to quit she/he shall be given assistance to do so. It is crucial that any major delay for the realisation is avoided as with time the motivational state of the patient is at risk.
Arrange	Follow-up is to be arranged to support success. The main goal is to avoid the risk of relapse and if relapse happens to help the patient to resume abstinence and stabilise it. Follow-up intervals must be adapted individually.

Table 1. Assessment of motivation and steps towards smoking cessation: The 5A-strategy [21].

Usually the first three steps ask/advise/assess are being applied repeatedly until finally the smoker might feel that his willingness to start action has reached the point.

The **5R-strategy** for patients unwilling to quit–"relevance, risk, rewards, roadblocks, repetition" (see **Table 2**) has shown to be helpful [25]. Using this, the 5R technique allows advancing an individual's state of readiness in quitting smoking, and strengthening their motivation to quit smoking.

Relevance: the relevance of quitting is discussed with the patient taking into account the individual health condition of the person.

Risk: the individual risk of the patient if continuing smoking is being made clear.

Rewards: the improvements of health conditions the patient can expect after quitting are discussed.

Roadblocks: barriers that hinder the smoker to take action are discussed in detail, for example, fear of withdrawal symptoms, fear of weight gaining etc.

Repetition: the strategy is to be performed repeatedly at every encounter with a smoker.

It has to be underlined that the main principles of the motivational interviewing technique shall be applied in the 5R-strategy. Among them, maintaining the smoker's autonomy may be the most important: pushing the patient towards any action must be avoided. Instead, all discussions shall be led following a pattern like "… if you as a smoker decided to quit: what might be the biggest advantage for you motivating you to do so …?"

3.3. Behavioural therapy

Behavioural therapy in various strategies is outlined as the main element of effective smoking cessation therapy [31, 32]. There is a strong dose-response relationship between the intensity of

Relevance	The relevance of quitting is discussed with the patient taking into account the individual health condition of the person. This means that the patient must be enabled to develop a clear understanding of his personal risks concerning his disease status which she/he shall understand clearly. Instruction must follow the intellectual capabilities of the patient.
Risk	The individual risk of the patient if continuing smoking is being made clear. Particularly for COPD patient, the course of her/his lung function loss with and without smoking respectively shall be made understood so the patient can understand how much her/his prognosis depends on successful quitting.
Rewards	The improvements of health conditions and life conditions the patient can expect after quitting are discussed. This includes short-term advantages like better exercise capabilities and less bronchitis symptoms within weeks as well as long-term rewards like longevity and overall performance improvement in later years. It also includes non-health advantages like saved money, better cosmetic appearance, being a better example for own children, gaining autonomy while losing dependence on nicotine etc.
Roadblocks	Barriers that hinder the smoker to take action are discussed in detail, for example, fear of withdrawal symptoms, fear of weight gaining etc. The therapist will ask the patient to find her/his own strategies to overcome the individual roadblocks of the particular patient by asking him to develop own personal solutions.
Repetition	The strategy is to be performed repeatedly at every encounter with a smoker. It is essential to focus on the necessity of abstinence at every meeting with the patient. Failure to bring the patient to action in one meeting is not a failure of the strategy. The repeated focusing on quitting by itself increases the patient ambivalence thus facilitating the development of eventual motivation towards action.

Table 2. The 5R-strategy for patients unwilling to quit [25].

tobacco dependence counselling and its effectiveness [33]. Interventions are designed to meet the smoker's limited willingness to take part in specific interventions on one hand and the knowledge that "the more the better" intervention should be intense with frequent days and long follow-up on the other hand. Successful interventions for smoking cessation group therapy are mostly restricted to 3–6 dates within 2–6 weeks with a total duration of about 10 hours. Programs following similar conception achieve abstinence rates of 30–45% after 12 months [34–37]. Behavioural therapy for smoking cessation includes psychoeducation aiming to establish a clear understanding of the necessity of quitting to stop negative effects mainly on health. Participants are being enabled to identify their personal smoking trigger situations and to develop alternative strategies to avoid smoking. This is done by explicitly increasing the ambivalence of the addicted smoker as to short-term smoking associated advantages in contrast to long-term disadvantages and risks. Participants receive support for preparation of their smoke stop day with detailed planning of the individual realisation. Participants receive detailed preparation for management of relapse risk situations and are being enabled for alternative strategies to avoid relapse. While there is a correlation of abstinence rates and intensity/duration of behavioural intervention, patients frequently are reluctant to accept longer behavioural interventions with multiple dates due to limitations from their daily life [38].

3.4. Pharmacotherapy

Pharmacotherapy can support smoking cessation therapy in patients with higher degrees of nicotine addiction and thus increase abstinence rates [39]. To measure total nicotine withdrawal discomfort or craving, various scales may be used [40]. The major underlying mechanism for increased abstinence rates with pharmacotherapy support consists in the continued partial saturation of nicotine specific receptors ($\alpha4\beta2$ receptors) in the ventral tegmental area of the brain allowing to maintain dopaminergic activity. Under this protection regarding the direct nicotine addiction proportion of tobacco dependence, the behavioural changes towards abstinence are facilitated while the exposition to toxic components of cigarette smoke is ended.

3.5. Nicotine replacement therapy

Nicotine replacement therapy [41] is longest established in support of smoking cessation therapy. Various OTC applications are available. Dosage should be planned following the smoking consumption amount at the time of the smoke stop. Roughly, smoking one cigarette results in the uptake of about 2 mg of nicotine for the smoker. Given, a smoker's consumption is 20 cigarettes a day, the replacement at the start of the measure should be roughly 40 mg. The composition of replacement products may be a basic application of a patch and addition of gums, lozenges or parts of oral nicotine spray to reach the amount. Side effects of nicotine replacement therapy are mostly restricted to irritability/impairment of sleep and sometimes local skin irritation (patches). Due to impaired teeth conditions, gums may not be applied properly. There is no evidence that NRT increases the risk of heart attacks [42, 43]. The toxic lethal dose of nicotine will not be reached by far due to the short half-time of nicotine.

3.6. Varenicline

Varenicline as a partial agonist and partial antagonist of the nicotine receptor was introduced for tobacco cessation therapy ever since 2006 first in the USA and then stepwise worldwide. The substance was suspected to cause depression and suicidal thinking and irritability as a side effect. Eventually studies could show, but those effects appeared due to withdrawal symptoms and could not be attributed to varenicline. The substance has turned out to be the most effective and save support of smoking cessation in various studies [44–46]. Varenicline is applied as tablets to be taken twice daily. Due to nausea as a possible side effect dosage is started with 0.5 mg twice daily to be continued with 1 mg twice daily over 3 months. Varenicline is to be started about 1 week before the planned quit day. Abnormal dreams and disturbed sleep are the main reported side effects both disappearing after the end of the application [47]. While varenicline was suspected to cause psychiatric side effects like irritability, depression and suicidal tendencies in the past, recent studies could show those effects as withdrawal effects. Former possible contraindication in psychiatric/schizophrenic patients are not maintained [46].

3.7. Bupropione

Bupropione was originally developed as an antidepressant but showed effects in supporting smoking cessation therapy. Due to possible side effects (lowered seizure threshold) and lower effectivity compared to other substances (varenicline etc.), it has now a minor role rather restricted to patients with depression in smoking cessation but may be taken into consideration for patients with depression [48].

4. Challenges to smoking cessation in COPD

4.1. Abstinence rates

Depending on the measures taken in tobacco cessation therapy, abstinence rates after 12 months can vary from about 3% over baseline after short advice to stop smoking up to nearly 50% following combined behavioural therapy and pharmacotherapy in an intensive setting [49–54].

4.2. Degree of addiction

COPD patients have higher dependence on tobacco [55, 56]. Higher dependence scores require not only a more intense behavioural therapy with more face-to-face contacts [38] and the possibility of individual psychotherapy if needed but also longer and more consequent application of pharmaceutical support. For example, the application duration of varenicline may be prolonged in patients with late relapse [57].

4.3. Role of depression

COPD patients have a higher depression rate [56, 58–63] COPD patients with depression require special treatment which takes specific depressed condition and consideration. In patients with a non-controlled depression, treatment of the depression is ranking before smoking cessation. Only after successful re-compensation of the psychiatric disease, the start of the cessation therapy should be undertaken [64–68].

4.4. Role of reimbursement

Reimbursement of tobacco cessation measures–regardless of the fact that a smoker who quits will save considerable sums of money and thus might pay for the cessation intervention–has shown to increase willingness to take part and to increase abstinence rates. It has to be accepted that addicted smokers have a different perception on spending considerable proportions of their income on tobacco products. Also, the major proportion of addicted smokers is a part of the less affluent and often has difficulties to pay for smoking cessation measures/medication at the given time when saving money with abstinence later [64, 65, 68].

4.5. Weight gain concerns

Minor weight gain after quitting average tobacco consumption is to be expected but can be avoided with higher physical activity [69–73]. Smoking one cigarette induces a loss of metabolic energy of about 10 kcal. Thus, a person who formerly smoked 20 cigarettes per day and who continues usual diet as before will have an increase of available energy of about 200 kcal per day after quitting. This results in a weight gain of about 5–7%. The person should be encouraged to accept this weight gain for a limited period of time until she/he will be a well-established secure ex-smoker with minimised relapse risk. It should be avoided to perform a weight control strategy while quitting as the success of the final abstinence, would be at risk with a double stress of smoking cessation and weight control efforts [70–72, 74].

4.6. Professional setting

The professional frame of tobacco cessation measures like behavioural therapy and pharmacotherapy counselling has a marked influence on long-time abstinence rates. Performing tobacco cessation therapy in physician practices as an integrated part of continuous therapy of their underlying disease appears to have a positive effect on long-time abstinence. This may be attributed to the fact that in the practice or outpatient ambulance, the patient will be seen after ending cessation therapy and continuously be monitored for maintaining abstinence, thus expecting specific questions from the physician who treats him. This may reduce relapse probability [54, 75, 76].

5. Role of e-cigarette

The e-cigarette is being introduced progressively as a possible instrument on the way to tobacco cessation and/or a measure of harm reduction respectively [77–79]. Increasing evidence appears to show that the e-cigarette may be helpful in smoking cessation particularly if containing a sufficient amount of nicotine which by itself does no harm to the respiratory system [78, 80].

Cell culture and experimental animal data indicate that e-cigs have the potential for inducing inflammation, albeit much less than smoking [81]. Evidence on possible hazards from e-cigarettes show increasingly clear that compared to tobacco cigarettes the risk of consumption of e-cigarettes is much less [82], while further research on the subject is on-going and necessary [83]. Recent research could show exposure to toxic and carcinogenic substances significantly lower in users of e-cigarettes as compared to cigarette smokers [77]. The FDA now has regulatory authority over e-cigs and can regulate product and e-liquid design features, such as nicotine content and delivery, voltage, e-liquid formulations and flavours. For patients who show no realistic willingness or ability of quitting and who in particular are not willing to apply nicotine replacement therapy products, the alternative of using E-cigarettes can be taken into consideration. Mainly two major potential risks of e-cigarette are being discussed at present. E-cigarettes might lead the consumer—mostly adolescents—into a tobacco cigarette consumer career, thus inducing possible lifelong addiction. E-cigarettes might contain compounds that might cause lung cancer although at a lower risk than tobacco cigarettes do. Both concerns hardly apply for COPD patients in far progressed stages of the disease where respiratory function by itself is acutely at risk. In particular for these COPD patients with highest degree of loss of lung function, the main goal must be to urgently avoid any further contact of toxic tobacco smoke with the bronchi. However, a great proportion of COPD patients in this situation due to their mental capacities and their addiction are not willing or able to avoid cigarette smoke by simply applying nicotine replacement as they will not be able to change their smoking habits which they feel can be preserved by using the e-cigarette. Thus, the goal of avoiding toxic smoke may be achieved by the application of e-cigarette vapour instead of tobacco smoke with high content of toxic and carcinogenic components. With more legal regulations on e-cigarette products worldwide and with a growing body of evidence on the toxic and carcinogenic potential, the role in smoking cessation/harm reduction will become clearer.

6. Summary

Smoking is the major cause of COPD resulting in respiratory impairment and increased mortality. Smoking cessation is the single effective intervention to mitigate the development of COPD. Most smokers are addicted to cigarettes, thus lacking control of consumption and ability to quit. Standardised motivation strategies in use elevated rates of willingness for smokers to consider quitting. High abstinence rates can be achieved by combination of behavioural therapy and pharmaceutical support. Medications to support behavioural therapy are effective and safe. Reimbursement of smoking cessation measures increases willingness and abstinence rates, where smoking cessation is not a realistic option patient with end-stage COPD, may benefit from the use of e-cigarette.

Author details

Thomas Hering[1,2,3,4,*]

*Address all correspondence to: hering@lungenarztpraxis-tegel.de

1 Lungenarztpraxis Tegel, Berlin, Germany

2 German Society for Pulmonology (DGP), Germany

3 Scientific Action Group for Tobacco Cessation (WAT), Germany

4 Federal Association of Pulmonologists (BDP), Germany

References

[1] Brody JS, Spira A. State of the art. Chronic obstructive pulmonary disease, inflammation, and lung cancer. Proceedings of the American Thoracic Society. 2006;**3**(6):535-537

[2] Saetta M. Airway inflammation in chronic obstructive pulmonary disease. American Journal of Respiratory and Critical Care Medicine. 1999;**160**(5 Pt 2):S17-S20

[3] Anthonisen NR, Connett JE, Murray RP. Smoking and lung function of lung health study participants after 11 years. American Journal of Respiratory and Critical Care Medicine. 2002;**166**(5):675-679

[4] de-Torres JP et al. Lung cancer in patients with chronic obstructive pulmonary disease. Development and validation of the COPD Lung Cancer Screening Score. American Journal of Respiratory and Critical Care Medicine. 2015;**191**(3):285-291

[5] Young RP et al. COPD prevalence is increased in lung cancer, independent of age, sex and smoking history. The European Respiratory Journal. 2009;**34**(2):380-386

[6] Habraken JM et al. Health-related quality of life in end-stage COPD and lung cancer patients. Journal of Pain and Symptom Management. 2009;**37**(6):973-981

[7] Chapman S, MacKenzie R. The global research neglect of unassisted smoking cessation: Causes and consequences. PLoS Medicine. 2010;**7**(2):e1000216

[8] West R, Sohal T. "Catastrophic" pathways to smoking cessation: Findings from national survey. BMJ. 2006;**332**(7539):458-460

[9] Lozano R et al. Global and regional mortality from 235 causes of death for 20 age groups in 1990 and 2010: A systematic analysis for the Global Burden of Disease Study 2010. Lancet. 2012;**380**(9859):2095-2128

[10] Vos T et al. Years lived with disability (YLDs) for 1160 sequelae of 289 diseases and injuries 1990-2010: A systematic analysis for the Global Burden of Disease Study 2010. Lancet. 2012;**380**(9859):2163-2196

[11] Tockman MS, Comstock GW. Respiratory risk factors and mortality: Longitudinal studies in Washington County, Maryland. The American Review of Respiratory Disease. 1989;**140**(3 Pt 2):S56-S63

[12] Burrows B et al. Quantitative relationships between cigarette smoking and ventilatory function. The American Review of Respiratory Disease. 1977;**115**(2):195-205

[13] Dransfield MT et al. Racial and gender differences in susceptibility to tobacco smoke among patients with chronic obstructive pulmonary disease. Respiratory Medicine. 2006;**100**(6, 6):1110

[14] Prescott E et al. Gender difference in smoking effects on lung function and risk of hospitalization for COPD: Results from a Danish longitudinal population study. The European Respiratory Journal. 1997;**10**(4):822-827

[15] Burney P, Jarvis D, Perez-Padilla R. The global burden of chronic respiratory disease in adults. The International Journal of Tuberculosis and Lung Disease. 2015;**19**(1):10-20

[16] Croghan IT et al. Gender differences among smokers receiving interventions for tobacco dependence in a medical setting. Addict Behav. 2009;**34**(1):61-67

[17] Mannino DM et al. Low lung function and incident lung cancer in the United States: Data from the first National Health and Nutrition Examination Survey follow-up. Archives of Internal Medicine. 2003;**163**(12):1475-1480

[18] Tockman MS et al. Airways obstruction and the risk for lung cancer. Annals of Internal Medicine. 1987;**106**(4):512-518

[19] Hopkins RJ et al. Reduced expiratory flow rate among heavy smokers increases lung cancer risk. Results from the National Lung Screening Trial-American College of Radiology Imaging Network Cohort. Annals of the American Thoracic Society. 2017;**14**(3):392-402

[20] Bae K et al. Severity of pulmonary emphysema and lung cancer: Analysis using quantitative lobar emphysema scoring. Medicine (Baltimore). 2016;**95**(48):e5494

[21] Zhong Y et al. Immediate consequences of cigarette smoking: rapid formation of polycyclic aromatic hydrocarbon diol epoxides. Chem Res Toxicol. 2011;**24**(2):246-252

[22] Hering T. Smoking cessation with COPD – Which effects are to be expected? Atemw.-Lungenkrkh. 2010;**Jahrgang 36**(Nr. 11/2010):454-459

[23] Anthonisen NR et al. The effects of a smoking cessation intervention on 14.5-year mortality: A randomized clinical trial. Annals of Internal Medicine. 2005;**142**(4):233-239

[24] Etter JF. Short-term change in self-reported COPD symptoms after smoking cessation in an internet sample. The European Respiratory Journal. 2010;**35**(6):1249-1255

[25] Clinical Practice Guideline Treating Tobacco U et al. A clinical practice guideline for treating tobacco use and dependence: 2008 update. A U.S. Public Health Service report. Am J Prev Med. 2008;**35**(2):158-176

[26] van Eerd EA et al. Smoking cessation for people with chronic obstructive pulmonary disease. Cochrane Database of Systematic Reviews. 2016;(8):CD010744.

[27] Lai DT et al. Motivational interviewing for smoking cessation. Cochrane Database of Systematic Reviews. 2010;(1):CD006936

[28] Rennard SI, Daughton DM. Smoking cessation. Chest. 2000;**117**(5 Suppl 2):360S-364S

[29] Solberg LI et al. Patient satisfaction and discussion of smoking cessation during clinical visits. Mayo Clinic Proceedings. 2001;**76**(2):138-143

[30] Barzilai DA et al. Does health habit counseling affect patient satisfaction? Preventive Medicine. 2001;**33**(6):595-599

[31] Ramon JM, Bruguera E. Real world study to evaluate the effectiveness of varenicline and cognitive-behavioural interventions for smoking cessation. International Journal of Environmental Research and Public Health. 2009;**6**(4):1530-1538

[32] Lancaster T, Stead LF. Individual behavioural counselling for smoking cessation. Cochrane Database of Systematic Reviews. 2005;(2):CD001292

[33] Fiore M, Jaén CR, et al. A clinical practice guideline for treating tobacco use and dependence: A US Public Health Service report. The Tobacco Use and Dependence Clinical Practice Guideline Panel, Staff, and Consortium Representatives. JAMA. 2000;**283**(24):3244-3254

[34] Batra A, Buchkremer G. Nichtrauchen! Erfolgreich aussteigen in sechs Schritten. 3. Auflage ed. Stuttgart: Kohlhammer; 2011

[35] Nowak M, C. Kröger. Das Rauchfrei Programm–Jahresevaluation. 2010. www.rauchfrei-programm.de, 2011.

[36] Hering T et al. Real-Life Evaluation of the Compact Program for Smoking Cessation. Pneumologie 2015;**69**(10):577-582

[37] Hering T et al. Real-Life-Evaluation des Kompakt-Programmes zur Tabakentwohnung. Pneumologie. 2015;**69**(10):577-582

[38] Mottillo S et al. Behavioural interventions for smoking cessation: A meta-analysis of randomized controlled trials. European Heart Journal. 2008

[39] Hering T. Modern medical support for smoking cessation. Internist (Berl). 2008

[40] West R et al. Assessing DSM-IV nicotine withdrawal symptoms: A comparison and evaluation of five different scales. Psychopharmacology. 2006;**184**(3-4):619-627

[41] Moore D et al. Effectiveness and safety of nicotine replacement therapy assisted reduction to stop smoking: Systematic review and meta-analysis. BMJ. 2009;**338**:b1024

[42] Stead LF et al. Nicotine replacement therapy for smoking cessation. Cochrane Database of Systematic Reviews. 2012;**11**:CD000146

[43] Benowitz NL, Gourlay SG. Cardiovascular toxicity of nicotine: Implications for nicotine replacement therapy. Journal of the American College of Cardiology. 1997;**29**(7):1422-1431

[44] Cahill K et al. Nicotine receptor partial agonists for smoking cessation. Cochrane Database of Systematic Reviews. 2016;**5**:CD006103

[45] Jimenez-Ruiz C, Berlin I, Hering T. Varenicline: A novel pharmacotherapy for smoking cessation. Drugs. 2009;**69**(10):1319-1338

[46] Anthenelli RM et al. Neuropsychiatric safety and efficacy of varenicline, bupropion, and nicotine patch in smokers with and without psychiatric disorders (EAGLES): A double-blind, randomised, placebo-controlled clinical trial. Lancet. 2016;**387**(10037):2507-2520

[47] Jimenez-Ruiz C, Hering T, Berlin I. Varenicline: A novel pharmacotherapy for smoking cessation. Drugs. 2009;**69**(10):1319-1338

[48] Hughes JR, Stead LF, Lancaster T. Antidepressants for smoking cessation. Cochrane Database of Systematic Reviews. 2007;**1**:CD000031

[49] Hughes JR, Keely J, Naud S. Shape of the relapse curve and long-term abstinence among untreated smokers. Addiction. 2004;**99**(1):29-38

[50] Piper ME et al. Gender, race, and education differences in abstinence rates among participants in two randomized smoking cessation trials. Nicotine & Tobacco Research. 2010;**12**(6):647-657

[51] Chatkin JM et al. Abstinence rates and predictors of outcome for smoking cessation: Do Brazilian smokers need special strategies? Addiction. 2004;**99**(6):778-784

[52] Murphy DB et al. Short-term and long-term abstinence rates associated with a hospital-based behavioral approach to smoking cessation. American Journal of Health Promotion. 1994;**8**(6):420-1, 424

[53] Manchon Walsh P et al. Effects of partner smoking status and gender on long term abstinence rates of patients receiving smoking cessation treatment. Addictive Behaviors. 2007;**32**(1):128-136

[54] Hering T et al. Real-Life Evaluation of the Compact Program for Smoking Cessation. Pneumologie. 2015;**69**(10):577-582

[55] Thabane M, C.W. Group. Smoking cessation for patients with chronic obstructive pulmonary disease (COPD): An evidence-based analysis. Ontario Health Technology Assessment Series. 2012;**12**(4):1-50

[56] Hill K et al. Anxiety and depression in end-stage COPD. The European Respiratory Journal. 2008;**31**(3):667-677

[57] Tonstad S et al. Effect of maintenance therapy with varenicline on smoking cessation: A randomized controlled trial. JAMA. 2006;**296**(1):64-71

[58] Ng TP et al. Co-morbid association of depression and COPD: A population-based study. Respiratory Medicine. 2009;**103**(6):895-901

[59] Korhonen T et al. Smoking behaviour as a predictor of depression among Finnish men and women: A prospective cohort study of adult twins. Psychological Medicine. 2006;1-11

[60] Hughes JR. Depression during tobacco abstinence. Nicotine & Tobacco Research. 2007;**9**(4): 443-446

[61] Wilson I. Depression in the patient with COPD. International Journal of Chronic Obstructive Pulmonary Disease. 2006;**1**(1):61-64

[62] Stage KB et al. Depression in COPD--management and quality of life considerations. International Journal of Chronic Obstructive Pulmonary Disease. 2006;**1**(3):315-320

[63] Schneider C et al. COPD and the risk of depression. Chest. 2010;**137**(2):341-347

[64] Tremblay M, Payette Y, Montreuil A. Use and reimbursement costs of smoking cessation medication under the Quebec public drug insurance plan. Canadian Journal of Public Health. 2009;**100**(6):417-420

[65] Twardella D, Brenner H. Effects of practitioner education, practitioner payment and reimbursement of patients' drug costs on smoking cessation in primary care: A cluster randomised trial. Tobacco Control. 2007;**16**(1):15-21

[66] Bertram MY et al. Costs and benefits of smoking cessation aids: Making a case for public reimbursement of nicotine replacement therapy in Australia. Tobacco Control. 2007;**16**(4):255-260

[67] Petersen R et al. Medicaid reimbursement for prenatal smoking intervention influences quitting and cessation. Tobacco Control. 2006;**15**(1):30-34

[68] Kaper J et al. Reimbursement for smoking cessation treatment may double the abstinence rate: Results of a randomized trial. Addiction. 2005;**100**(7):1012-1020

[69] Parsons AC et al. Interventions for preventing weight gain after smoking cessation. Cochrane Database of Systematic Reviews. 2009;**1**:CD006219

[70] O'Hara P et al. Early and late weight gain following smoking cessation in the Lung Health Study. American Journal of Epidemiology. 1998;**148**(9):821-830

[71] Hall SM et al. Weight gain prevention and smoking cessation: Cautionary findings. American Journal of Public Health. 1992;**82**(6):799-803

[72] Williamson DF et al. Smoking cessation and severity of weight gain in a national cohort. The New England Journal of Medicine. 1991;**324**(11):739-745

[73] Williamson DF et al. The 10-year incidence of overweight and major weight gain in US adults. Archives of Internal Medicine. 1990;**150**(3):665-672

[74] Swan GE, Carmelli D. Characteristics associated with excessive weight gain after smoking cessation in men. American Journal of Public Health. 1995;**85**(1):73-77

[75] Tottenborg SS et al. Determinants of smoking cessation in patients with COPD treated in the outpatient setting. Chest. 2016;**150**(3):554-562

[76] Hering T et al. Smoking cessation in pneumological routine care. Pneumologie. 2011;**65**(11): 692-696

[77] Shahab L et al. Nicotine, Carcinogen, and Toxin Exposure in Long-Term E-Cigarette and Nicotine Replacement Therapy Users: A Cross-sectional Study. Ann Intern Med. 2017;**166**(6):390-400

[78] Hajek P et al. Nicotine delivery to users from cigarettes and from different types of e-cigarettes. Psychopharmacology (Berl). 2017;**234**(5):773-779

[79] McNeill A et al. E-cigarettes: An Evidence Update–A Report Commissioned by Public Health England. 2015

[80] Hartmann-Boyce J et al. Electronic cigarettes for smoking cessation. Cochrane Database of Systematic Reviews. 2016;**9**:CD010216

[81] Shields PG et al. A Review of Pulmonary Toxicity of Electronic Cigarettes in the Context of Smoking: A Focus on Inflammation. Cancer Epidemiol Biomarkers Prev. 2017;**26**(8):1175-1191

[82] Royal_College_of_Physicians. Nicotine Without Smoke: Tobacco Harm Reduction. 2016. www.rcplondon.ac.uk

[83] El Dib R et al. Electronic nicotine delivery systems and/or electronic non-nicotine delivery systems for tobacco smoking cessation or reduction: A systematic review and meta-analysis. BMJ Open. 2017;**7**(2):e012680

Chapter 6

Pulmonary Rehabilitation in COPD: Current Practice and Future Directions

Michelle Casey, Amy Mulkerns,
Cliona O'Donnell and Tim McDonnell

Additional information is available at the end of the chapter

http://dx.doi.org/10.5772/intechopen.71218

Abstract

This chapter will review the rationale for and the need for pulmonary rehabilitation in patients with Chronic Obstructive Pulmonary Disease (COPD). Its clinical effectiveness will be considered, including the evidence supporting a role for rehabilitation in improving exercise tolerance in COPD as measured. While the influence of pulmonary rehabilitation on dyspnoea, exercise tolerance and quality-of-life is clear, evidence for the benefits of rehabilitation on reducing healthcare utilisation such as admission to hospital or attendance at out-of-hours services is limited. The chapter will provide guidance on the setting up of a pulmonary rehabilitation programme and clinical staff required and the suitability of patients to enter such programmes will be outlined. There will be discussion on the key components of a programme including education, nutritional advice and the management of dyspnoea. Exercise is the central component of pulmonary rehabilitation. Assessment of the patient and prescription of an exercise programme will be outlined as will assessing a patient's improvement. One key goal of pulmonary rehabilitation is ongoing lifestyle modification to encourage patients to undertake a more active lifestyle in the future. Ways of activating patients to do this will be discussed and the evidence for the use of telehealth in this area will be reviewed.

Keywords: pulmonary rehabilitation, COPD, exercise, physical activity

1. Introduction

COPD is a systemic disease associated with extra pulmonary effects such as osteopaenia, muscle wasting, cardiovascular disease and depression [1]. The symptoms of COPD make engagement in physical activity unpleasant. Air trapping and hyperinflation of the lungs cause increased breathlessness due to the resultant inefficient breathing. The breathlessness itself provokes anxiety, which in turn leads to further breathlessness, exacerbations of COPD and episodes of panic. Due to this, activities that involve physical exertion are avoided, leading to muscle deconditioning and a further reduced capacity to engage in physical activity. Pulmonary rehabilitation improves symptoms, quality of life and health-care utilisation in patients with COPD [1, 2].

Pulmonary rehabilitation is defined as "an interdisciplinary programme of care for patients with chronic respiratory impairment that is individually tailored and designed to optimise each patient's physical and social performance and autonomy. Programmes comprise individualised exercise programmes and education" [3]. Physical inactivity is a key predictor of mortality in COPD and consequently all major guidelines highlight the importance of exercise in the treatment and management of COPD. There is now high quality evidence for improved exercise capacity, health-related quality of life and decreased breathlessness, fatigue and health-care utilisation following pulmonary rehabilitation [1].

Pulmonary rehabilitation is focussed on an interdisciplinary and holistic approach to the management of COPD, emphasising behavioural change as a key component. It fits very well with the concept of integrated care, with its cornerstone being individually tailored exercise training. Patient assessment, education, psychosocial support and nutritional counselling are also included in the standard pulmonary rehabilitation programme. Overall, the focus of a pulmonary rehabilitation programme is to alleviate the physiological effects of the disease process and decrease the psychosocial effects of the illness on the individual.

2. Historical development

The effects of exercise in patients with chronic respiratory diseases have been a subject for study for some time. By the middle of the 20th century, accepted wisdom was that dyspnoea on exertion should be avoided [4]. Dr. Alvan Barach was the first to offer a contrary opinion in the 1950s, with his advice to "remember to cure the patient as well as the disease". Thomas L. Petty was the first to establish an out-patient programme of pulmonary rehabilitation in the 1960s, despite the conventional wisdom of not exerting patients with respiratory limitations. This programme included individualised instruction, bronchial hygiene, breathing retraining, physical reconditioning and individualised pharmacologic therapy. Rehabilitation programmes were set up throughout the USA, and Petty noted improved exercise tolerance, reduced hospitalisations and a return to gainful employment in the majority of his patients [4]. Subsequently, in the 1980s a view became prevalent that as exercise conditioning did not improve lung function, pulmonary rehabilitation was unlikely to provide physiological benefit to patients. It was felt that if physiological benefit was not demonstrated, the programme design was not particularly important. Finally, in the 1990s, physiologic benefit was proven by using exercise at a higher intensity and the concept of pulmonary rehabilitation was reinvigorated [4, 5].

3. Rationale for pulmonary rehabilitation

Pulmonary rehabilitation is designed to reduce the symptoms of COPD, improve health related quality of life (HRQoL), improve and re-establish functional ability, enhance participation in everyday life and promote patient autonomy. The exercise component of pulmonary rehabilitation increases inspiratory volume and reduces dynamic hyperinflation, both of which reduce dyspnoea when a person is performing tasks. Exercise also increases muscle function, which delays fatigue and results in increased exercise tolerance. The educational component focuses on self-management and behaviour change. Providing information and knowledge, skills such as goal setting, problem solving and decision making, along with action plans to better recognise and manage their disease are all integral parts of the programme. Modifying nutritional intake and smoking patterns, medication adherence and utilising effective energy saving strategies and breathing techniques are part of the education component [1].

The exercise capacity of patients with COPD is often impaired and limited by dyspnoea. The reasons for this are complex and multifactorial, including defective gas exchange, dynamic hyperinflation, peripheral muscle dysfunction, respiratory muscle dysfunction, the effects of physical deconditioning, the presence of co-morbidities and the natural age-related decline in exercise capacity [6]. Physical exercise in pulmonary rehabilitation is the best method of improving muscle function and skeletal muscle adaption in patients with COPD [5, 7–10]. The benefits pulmonary rehabilitation produces are explained by improvements in muscle function and the oxidative capacity and efficiency of skeletal muscles, despite the absence of any changes in lung function [11, 12]. Other related improvements include increased motivation, improved mood and improved cardiovascular functioning, which result in ongoing participation in exercise beyond the rehabilitation programme [13].

Even those patients with severe chronic respiratory disease can often sustain the necessary training intensity and duration for skeletal muscle adaptation. Skeletal muscle adaptation following exercise training leads to gains in exercise capacity despite the absence of changes in lung function. In addition, the improved oxidative capacity and efficiency of the skeletal muscles leads to a reduced ventilator requirement for a given submaximal work rate. This could reduce dynamic hyperinflation, adding to the reduction in exertional dyspnoea [6]. Medical therapy should be optimised prior to exercise training beginning and a patient assessment is required prior to beginning an exercise programme.

4. The clinical effectiveness of pulmonary rehabilitation

4.1. Physiological

One of the first studies to show an improvement in exercise tolerance following exercise training in COPD was Casaburi et al. in 1991 [14]. They showed a statistically significant improvement in exercise tolerance and reduced blood lactate and ventilatory requirement post exercise. These findings have been supported by others [5] and a Cochrane review in 2009 [2] showed a statistically significant improvement in exercise capacity in people who underwent a pulmonary rehabilitation programme. Results of a further Cochrane review in 2015 strongly supported the benefits of pulmonary rehabilitation [1]. They found clinically and statistically significant improvements in important domains of health-related quality of life, including dyspnoea, fatigue, emotional function and mastery, as well as the 6 minute walk test: a measure of functional exercise [1]. Also noted was a small but statistically significant improvement in physical activity levels. Physical activity has become more important in COPD management as it has been shown that inactivity is linked with reduced survival, poorer quality of life and increased healthcare utilisation [15].

4.2. Quality of life

The benefits of pulmonary rehabilitation on dyspnoea and health status have been supported by a Cochrane review [1]. The Chronic Respiratory Questionnaire was used in a number of studies and showed an improvement in dyspnoea that was statistically significant and clinically relevant. Improvement was also noted in the other CRQ domains of fatigue, emotional function and patient's sense of control. The St. Georges Respiratory Questionnaire Scores were also subject to a meta-analysis in the same Cochrane review and found to show significant improvement following pulmonary rehabilitation [16].

4.3. Reduction of healthcare utilisation

Several studies have investigated whether pulmonary rehabilitation leads to a decrease in the number of caregiver or physician visits, hospital days, and medication use [3, 6]. In general, some benefit is shown in this important area. Several randomised studies comparing pulmonary rehabilitation with usual care found a trend towards reduced hospital admissions and hospital days. Studies comparing healthcare use before and after pulmonary rehabilitation show that pulmonary rehabilitation significantly reduced emergency room visits and physician visits [3, 6].

4.4. Psychosocial

In a Cochrane review published in 2015, participants allocated to rehabilitation had significantly greater changes in HRQoL [17]. A Cochrane review in 2009 had previously shown moderate to large effects of rehabilitation on health-related quality of life and exercise capacity [2].

4.5. Self-efficacy

Self-efficacy refers to the level of belief someone has in their ability to complete a chosen task or goal. Overall, self-efficacy scores improve with pulmonary rehabilitation [1].

4.6. Survival

There is limited evidence for increased survival to date, however only one randomised controlled trial has looked at survival: the control group received education and the intervention group received rehabilitation and education. The study was unlikely to be powered to detect mortality [18]. A prospective observational study of 1218 patients showed no mortality benefit from pulmonary rehabilitation [19]; however, another study did show improved mortality in patients where exercise capacity and dyspnoea improved after rehabilitation only [9].

4.7. Nutrition

In an underweight population, some small weight gain was noted following exercise training; however, in general the effect of pulmonary rehabilitation on nutritional status does not appear to be significant. Nutritional outcomes at the start of a rehabilitation programme do not affect outcomes such as exercise capacity or health status [6].

5. Setting up a pulmonary rehabilitation Programme

5.1. Duration

There remains no consensus internationally on the optimum duration of a pulmonary rehabilitation programme. However, pulmonary rehabilitation programmes of 6–12 weeks are recommended and demonstrate a significant benefit in health status, dyspnoea and exercise in patients with chronic respiratory diseases limited by breathlessness. An attendance at a minimum of 12 exercise sessions is recommended to successfully complete the programme. Programmes of less than 6 weeks have been shown to provide some benefits in health status and exercise capacity in individuals with COPD; however, these programmes should be individualised and measures of benefit should be in place prior to the patient concluding the programme. The ongoing benefits of a pulmonary rehabilitation programme of longer than 3 months duration has been shown, including changes in daily physical activity levels, but the cost benefit of these remains unclear [3, 6, 20–22].

5.2. Frequency

The recommended frequency of exercise classes also differs internationally. The general consensus supports a minimum of two supervised exercise sessions per week, and either a third supervised session or formalised unsupervised session depending on the resources available. This is in contrast with the WHO recommendation of 5 sessions of 30 minutes exercise per week. However, to date the key improvement outcomes in pulmonary rehabilitation are based on at least two supervised sessions per week. Pulmonary rehabilitation programmes should therefore encompass a minimum of twice weekly supervised exercise sessions, a third session of prescribed unsupervised exercise and encouragement of regular physical activity for 30 minutes five days per week in line with standard healthy living advice [3, 6, 20–22].

5.3. Staffing

There is no consensus on staffing levels for a pulmonary rehabilitation programme. The staffing of the programmes varies globally, with physical therapists coordinating programmes in Australia, South America and Europe, while respiratory therapists coordinate programmes in the United States. There is no one best staffing structure. Optimal staff-patient ratios also differ: the American Association of Cardiovascular and Pulmonary Rehabilitation recommends ratios of 1:4 for exercise training, 1:8 for educational sessions and 1:1 for complex patients; the British Thoracic Society recommends ratios of 1:8 for exercise training and 1:16 for educational sessions. These ratios are not evidence based and are designed based on experience and opinion [3, 6, 20–22].

It is recommended and accepted that for patients to gain optimum benefit from a pulmonary rehabilitation programme, a multidisciplinary approach should be taken [13, 23]. Availability of resources and staff will dictate the level of input the Multidisciplinary team will have but each member plays an important role in the rehabilitation programme:

- *Respiratory physician*: medical assessment; pharmacological management; referral; screening for oxygen and oxygen prescription.
- *Physiotherapist*: exercise testing, prescription and training; musculoskeletal assessment, treatment and advice; airway clearance education; strategies for the management of dyspnoea; inspiratory muscle training; assessment for ambulatory oxygen requirements.
- *Respiratory nurse*: Disease specific education; development of action plans; inhaler technique training.
- *Dietician*: Nutritional assessment and advice.
- *Occupational therapist*: Assessment and modification of home environment; energy conservation advice.
- *Pharmacist*: advice and education on respiratory education and inhaler use.
- *Social worker*: information and access to support services.
- *Psychologist:* psychosocial assessment and treatment for conditions including panic, anxiety and depression.

5.4. Rolling or cohort programme

Deciding on whether to administer a rolling or a cohort programme is dependent on local considerations, as there is no high-quality evidence to suggest the benefit of one over the other. The characteristics of a rolling and a cohort programme are outlined in **Table 1** [3]:

	Rolling	Cohort
Nature of programme	Continual cycle of sessions, where patients join when there is a space available and leave after completing the programme of sessions	All patients start and finish the programme at the same time
Waiting list	Patients enter the programme when a space arises, permits fast track access, potentially allows better capacity	An accumulative number of patients wait to start the programme, the waiting list may be distorted
Rehabilitation delivered at different locations by the same team	Not possible as the programme always runs in the same venue	Suitable
Education programme	The order of the talk is individual and governed by the point of entry	Can 'flow' in a logical order
Group dynamics	A new patient may be the sole new participant which may be a beneficial or a challenge	Patients all start together which permits group leaning of lifestyle changes
Assessments	Must perform pre and post assessments in parallel to the course	Dedicated assessment slots can be programmed for all subjects pre and post rehabilitation
Duration of programme	Allows lengthening the programme or early graduation as required	Fixed length for each programme

Table 1. Characteristics of Rolling and Cohort programmes.

5.5. Selection criteria for pulmonary rehabilitation programmes

Any person with a chronic lung condition who continues to be limited by breathlessness despite optimal medical management should be considered for a pulmonary rehabilitation programme [22]. Improvements following a pulmonary rehabilitation programme have been shown in patients with COPD irrespective of their age or gender [24–26] level of functional impairment [27–29] or disease severity [30, 31]. By promoting self-efficacy and behaviour change, improving exercise tolerance and physical activity and reducing exacerbations, pulmonary rehabilitation at an earlier stage of disease has the potential to markedly change the course of the disease [6]. Frequent reasons for referral to a pulmonary rehabilitation programme include:

- Dyspnoea/fatigue and chronic respiratory symptoms.
- Impaired health-related quality of life.
- Decreased functional status.
- Difficulty performing activities of daily living.
- Increased use of medical resources (e.g., frequent exacerbations, hospitalizations, emergency room visits).
- One of the primary indicators for referral to pulmonary rehabilitation is based on the modified Medical Research Council Breathlessness (mMRC) score (see **Table 2**) [3]. This scale

measures perceived respiratory disability, and allows patients to indicate the extent to which their breathlessness impacts their mobility. It is a 0–4 grade scale used to establish levels of perceived breathlessness [3, 6].

There is very strong evidence that patients with an mMRC dyspnoea score of 2–4 who are functionally limited by breathlessness should be referred for pulmonary rehabilitation. However, patients with an mMRC dyspnoea score of 1 who are functionally limited by breathlessness should also be referred for pulmonary rehabilitation. Patients with COPD who have an mMRC score of 4 but who are able to attend an outpatient pulmonary rehabilitation programme achieve similar benefits from the programme as those with a lower breathlessness score [28].

5.6. Exclusion criteria

The exclusion criteria for enrolment into a pulmonary rehabilitation programme are minimal, and in some cases participation in the programme by a patient can be facilitated by the attendance and support of a carer or relative. However, general exclusion guidelines would include [3, 6]:

- Patients with unstable cardiovascular disease or mobility problems which make exercising safely impossible (for example, severe arthritis, severe peripheral vascular disease, severe orthopaedic conditions).
- Patients with significant psychiatric or cognitive impairment who are unable to follow simple instructions safely in a group setting.
- Any further excluding factors are based on the assessor's own objective judgement or with a discussion with the referring physician, for example, a perceived lack of motivation to participate in the programme.

5.7. Referral process

Once a patient has been deemed suitable to attend a pulmonary rehabilitation programme by the healthcare professional, the referral should be used as an opportunity to educate the patient about the benefits of the programme, to explore their understanding of the programme

Grade	Degree of breathlessness related to activities
0	Not troubled by breathless except on strenuous exercise
1	Short of breath when hurrying or walking up a slight hill
2	Walks slower than contemporaries on level ground because of breathlessness or has to stop for breath when walking at own pace
3	Stops for breath after walking 100 metres or after a few minutes on level ground
4	Too breathless to leave the house, or breathless when dressing or undressing

Table 2. The modified Medical Research Council Breathlessness (mMRC) score.

and to address the patients' concerns [3]. The programme should be presented to the patient as a core treatment for the management of their condition as opposed to an optional adjunct. Patients should be referred to the programme under the care of a respiratory physician, who should be available to the staff co-ordinating the programme to discuss any medical problems which may arise during the programme and to ensure that potential participants have been medically assessed for suitability for the programme and that their pharmacological management has been optimised [22].

5.8. Pulmonary rehabilitation post exacerbations of COPD

Exacerbations of COPD result in increased mortality and healthcare use, worsening symptoms and health-related quality of life, as well as impaired exercise capacity, reduced skeletal muscle function of the lower limbs and reduced physical activity levels [3, 6]. Studies have therefore been conducted to explore the merits and the safety of 'early' pulmonary rehabilitation both during a hospital admission and within 1 month of hospital discharge for an acute exacerbation of COPD. It is now known that early pulmonary rehabilitation post exacerbation [2]:

- Is not associated with any adverse events or increased mortality
- Reduces risk of hospital readmissions
- Improves health related quality of life
- Improves exercise capacity

It is therefore recommended unequivocally that patients with COPD who are hospitalised for an acute exacerbation should be referred for pulmonary rehabilitation at discharge, and should be enrolled into the pulmonary rehabilitation programme within 1 month of leaving the hospital.

6. Patient assessment

The initial assessment for the programme is an opportunity to outline a detailed description of the programme to the patient, to assess for co-morbidities, risk factors and contraindications for the programme, and to consider any appropriate onward referrals to maximise the benefit the patient will receive from the programme [3]. The essential information required for pulmonary rehabilitation includes:

- Known communication/language barriers.
- Current activity levels.
- Respiratory diagnosis: spirometry for those with COPD.
- Height, weight, BP and oxygen saturations at rest are desirable.
- Modified Medical Research Council breathlessness score.

- Smoking status (for those who continue to smoke, document details of previous attempts to quit; recent quitters may require support and/or counselling).
- Therapies: current list of medication.
- Use of oxygen: long-term oxygen therapy, short-burst oxygen therapy, ambulatory; oxygen saturations, use of domiciliary Positive Pressure Ventilation.
- Significant and relevant comorbidities (which may affect their ability to participate in the exercise programme or education sessions, including adequacy of literacy and vision).
- Transport needs: if applicable to that rehabilitation provider.
- Health care utilisation: including number of hospital admissions and length of stay in the previous 12 months.

6.1. Specific situations at assessment

When deciding on a patient's suitability for pulmonary rehabilitation, there are certain groups of patient characteristics which need further consideration during assessment for the programme including [3]:

6.1.1. Smoking status

There is currently no evidence that smokers benefit any less from pulmonary rehabilitation than non-smokers, and the rehabilitation programme can be an ideal opportunity to support and facilitate these patients in smoking cessation. Smokers should be offered smoking cessation advice and should be referred to smoking cessation programmes.

6.1.2. Chronic respiratory failure

Patients with chronic respiratory failure ($PaO2 < 8$ kPa, $PO2 > 6$ kPa or both) gain much benefit from pulmonary rehabilitation and should not be excluded from the programme for this reason alone. The use of oxygen and non-invasive ventilation for these patients during the programme should be discussed with the referring physician, and the safety of the patient with consideration to the skill mix of the staff in the programme and the programme setting should also be considered when accepting these patients onto the programme.

6.1.3. Cardiovascular disease

From a safety perspective, patients with unstable cardiovascular disease (e.g. unstable angina, unstable arrhythmias) should not commence a pulmonary rehabilitation programme until their cardiac condition is stabilised. However, patients with stable cardiovascular disease as well as a chronic respiratory disease do benefit from the programme, and should be referred if pulmonary rehabilitation is indicated. Patients with aortic aneurysms <5.5 cm can participate safely in moderate intensity aerobic exercise training as long as their blood pressure is monitored and controlled.

http://dx.doi.org/10.5772/intechopen.71218

6.1.4. Anxiety and depression

Patients with symptoms of anxiety and depression also benefit from the pulmonary rehabilitation programme, and should not be excluded from referral to the programme. The pulmonary rehabilitation programme allows an opportunity to detect these conditions and to consider onward referral for optimal management.

6.1.5. Obese subjects

Pulmonary rehabilitation may be an ideal setting in which to address the needs of obese patients with associated respiratory symptoms, including exercise training, nutritional education, psychological support and onward referral to specialists as required. Obese patients should not be excluded from the pulmonary rehabilitation programme; however, assessments for other cardiac and pulmonary comorbidities may need to be considered prior to commencing the pulmonary rehabilitation programme. Weight limits of equipment should be considered, low impact exercises may be more appropriate and specialised equipment may be required to accommodate these patients [6].

6.1.6. Co-morbidities

COPD is commonly associated with other medical co-morbidities, which may result from the common risk factors for COPD such as smoking as well as systemic inflammation. These can further impact on the patient's management, and can include cardiovascular disease (arrhythmias, congestive heart failure, hypertension, and coronary disease), metabolic conditions (diabetes mellitus, osteoarthritis, and hyperlipidaemia), infections, lung cancer, obstructive sleep apnoea, cognitive dysfunction, depression or anxiety. These co-morbidities must be considered in the assessment and management of COPD patients enrolled in a pulmonary rehabilitation programme, as early intervention may influence the course and prognosis of the disease and can have a beneficial effect on both COPD and the relevant co-morbidity. Pulmonary rehabilitation is very important for patients with COPD and co-morbidities as physical activity is well documented to not only benefit COPD but also many other chronic conditions including obesity, diabetes, cardiovascular disease, musculoskeletal disease and peripheral vascular disease [32–36].

The presence of co-morbidities does not preclude pulmonary rehabilitation in patients with COPD but they should be considered thoroughly when monitoring and prescribing exercise to allow these individuals to exercise safely. For patients with cardiac conditions, the need for pre-rehabilitation investigations (for example, echocardiography or stress testing) should be discussed with the referring physician to define safe exercise parameters. Anaemia, orthopaedic and neurological issues require further consideration of a safe exercise plan and the need for specialised equipment. The patient may also require further onward referrals (for example, dual energy X-ray absorptiometry (DEXA) scan, psychological review, and nutritional review) based on observations during the exercise programme.

6.2. Exercise testing

Prior to commencing the rehabilitation programme, an exercise assessment is essential to [6]:

- Ensure the patient is safe to participate
- Rule out cardiovascular morbidities
- Assess baseline capacity
- Individualise exercise prescription
- Assess for the need for supplementary oxygen
- Define the factors contributing to exercise limitation
- Evaluate the effectiveness of the intervention

Exercise tests can include field walking tests, or laboratory cycle ergometer or treadmill tests. Field walking tests are most commonly used, and are considered more reflective of daily living; they are low cost and are convenient in most settings. These include the 6-minute walk test (6MWT) and the incremental shuttle walk test (ISWT). The 6MWT is a valid, reliable and reproducible self-paced walk test once the established, recommended and standardised protocol is used. Performed over a minimum of 30 metres, patients are asked to walk as far as possible in 6 minutes along a flat corridor [37]. The ISWT is a symptom limited maximal exercise capacity, externally paced walk test performed over a 10-metre course. It is also valid and reliable. The walk speed continues until the participant can no longer continue, with a maximum duration of 20 minutes. The endurance shuttle walks test (ESWT) is a constant walking speed test performed at a set speed based on the ISWT [6].

The choice of test is usually decided based on objectives, time, cost and availability.

7. Exercise training in pulmonary rehabilitation

Lower limb weakness is commonly seen in patients with COPD, and is a poor prognostic indicator [12]. The exercise component of pulmonary rehabilitation therefore should primarily be delivered reflecting aerobic exercise and on lower limb endurance and resistance training. The general principles of exercise in COPD are no different than in exercising a healthy population: it must reflect the individuals own capacity, progress as improvement occurs and exceed normal loads encountered in daily life to improve aerobic capacity and muscle strength.

7.1. Aerobic/endurance training

A target intensity of 60% peak work rate, aiming for an accumulative time of 30–60 minutes of aerobic training per session is recommended, with 30 minutes of continuous aerobic activity [3]. However, both interval and continuous training have been shown to be effective in patients with COPD, and should be selected based on both therapist and patient preference. Endurance exercise, most commonly delivered in the form of walking (treadmill or ground walking) or cycling, three to five times per week at a Borg dyspnoea or fatigue score of 4–6 (moderate to severe) is the recommended target training intensity [6].

7.2. Resistance training of the lower limbs

Resistance training of all major muscle groups, but particularly the quadriceps, should also be incorporated, not only for the improvements that are well documented for COPD symptoms, but also to reduce falls and to improve or maintain bone mineral density [6]. Resistance training should aim for 2–4 sets of 10–15 repetitions of each exercise, on 2–3 days of the week. The selected weight should be individualised for each patient, aiming for a prescribed weight of 60–70% of 1 repetition maximum for each individual patient. The weight should only have progressed once all sets can be completed with the selected weight [6]. Based on local resources, weight machines, elastic bands or free weights are all acceptable forms of resistance training.

7.3. Resistance training of the upper limbs

While it is suggested that upper limb training can improve upper limb function in patients with COPD, the optimal prescription of this training remains unclear, as do the improvements gained in broader outcomes for COPD patients. However, upper limb training may be incorporated based on individual needs to improve functional living. It could be assumed that starting loads and progression may follow the same prescription as for lower limb training [20].

7.4. Flexibility training

While minimal research has been done on flexibility training as part of the pulmonary rehabilitation programme or the optimal duration and intensity of stretching exercises, flexibility of the major upper and lower limb muscle groups on 2–3 days a week can be recommended [38]. Also, improved thoracic mobility and posture may improve vital capacity in COPD patients, and should be assessed and addressed in all COPD patients [6].

7.5. Generic vs. individualised exercise programmes

Generic exercise training is recommended for the pulmonary rehabilitation classes: all patients in the class should do all the same exercises as opposed to an individualised exercise programme for each patient. However, the prescription of exercise should be individualised to each patient to ensure the correct intensity for that patient. Goal setting should be addressed with each patient on the initial assessment to address any hurdles to exercise and to further address each patient's specific needs [3].

8. Education in pulmonary rehabilitation

Education on COPD and its management to both patient and family is an integral component of pulmonary rehabilitation programmes. Several studies show that patients instructed about the nature of their disease and the implications of therapy can better understand, recognise, and treat the symptoms of their disease [39]. The educational component acts as a support to lifestyle and behavioural change, and assists in the development of self-management skills. Patients are empowered to actively participate in their own healthcare, which can promote adherence to therapy and self-efficacy (i.e., the confidence in successfully managing one's health). The educational needs of each patient should be individualised and identified at the initial assessment and reassessed over the course of the programme. The style of teaching used in pulmonary rehabilitation is changing from traditional didactic lectures to a collaborative self-management approach, which may be more effective [6]. Education should run in conjunction with an exercise programme and should cover relevant topics associated with chronic lung disease. Different aspects should be delivered by different healthcare professionals involved in the programme, with the relevant expertise in that area.

Self-management includes core generic strategies, such as goal setting, problem solving, decision making, adherence to medication, maintaining regular exercise, nutritional advice, breathing techniques, bronchial hygiene and smoking cessation [40, 41]. Behavioural change strategies including the prevention, early recognition and treatment of exacerbations and advanced care directives are additional core educational issues incorporated in collaborative self-management programmes. The development of a patient-specific, collaborative self-management plan for COPD exacerbations including the recognition of symptoms, a personalised action plan and communication with a healthcare provider has been shown to be beneficial [41, 42].

8.1. Breathing strategies

Breathing strategies encompasses a range of breathing techniques, including active expiration, pursed lip breathing, diaphragmatic breathing, adapting certain body positions and co-ordinating paced breathing with activities. The aim of these techniques is to improve regional ventilation, gas exchange, respiratory muscle function, dyspnoea, exercise tolerance and quality of life [43].

The breathing strategies are tailored to the individual, with patients adopting the technique most effective in reducing symptoms [44].

8.2. Bronchial hygiene techniques

Excessive airway secretions secondary to mucus hypersecretion and impaired mucociliary clearance are distinctive features for some patients. Chest physiotherapy is used to aid removal of airway secretions, which involves teaching on importance of daily clearance and training in drainage techniques [45].

8.3. Smoking cessation

In approximately 90% of cases of COPD, cigarette smoking is the direct cause. The single most important intervention to retard the progression of air-flow limitation and improve survival is smoking cessation. For many patients smoking cessation may be difficult due to strong physiologic and psychological dependence. Long-term quit success rates of up to 25% can be achieved when sufficient reserves and time are dedicated to smoking cessation programmes [46]. The rehabilitation programme provides a forum for education and continued reinforcement, on risks of continued smoking, advice on nicotine replacement therapy and other pharmacotherapy, along with referral to smoking cessation programmes.

8.4. Advance care planning

The process of advance care planning is often inadequate in chronic respiratory diseases [47]. Anxiety and fear of death is well described in individuals with advanced COPD along with reluctance to discuss it with their treating physician [48]. The pulmonary rehabilitation programme has been identified as an appropriate setting for discussion on advance care planning and end of life care [49].

The idea is to allow both patient and family a unique opportunity to communicate goals of treatment and preferences regarding the use of life-sustaining treatments, such as cardiopulmonary resuscitation, mechanical ventilation, dialysis and feeding tubes, with the health care provider. Ideally, the discussion will facilitate better understanding of certain topics, such as the disease itself and prognosis, process of dying and end-of life care, advance directive documents (e.g. designating a health care proxy or enduring power of attorney).

8.5. Psychosocial support

Severe COPD is associated with increased risk for anxiety and depression, which can affect motivation levels and result in decreased participation in social activities [6, 46]. Episodes of dyspnoea often trigger fear and anxiety in patients with COPD and result in further anxiety in anticipation of repeat episodes [50]. Depression, feelings of hopelessness and an inability to cope are common in patients with COPD, with an approximate prevalence rate of 45% in patients with moderate to severe disease [51, 52]. Patients with depression have the tendency to withdraw from social interactions which can worsen feelings of isolation and loneliness. Sexual activity can be affected by depression and also the physical restrictions imposed by COPD itself, sexuality should be raised and discussed when necessary and appropriate counselling initiated.

Screening for anxiety and depression should be included at the initial assessment in a pulmonary rehabilitation programme. If possible interviewing and involving the caregiver is beneficial. Promotion of an adequate patient support system is an important component of pulmonary rehabilitation [53]. Psychological and social support provided within the pulmonary rehabilitation setting can facilitate adjustment the physiological impact of the disease by encouraging adaptive thoughts and behaviours. These aid patients in diminishing negative emotions, provides a socially supportive environment and may improve compliance with rehabilitation. Multidisciplinary team members with the appropriate expertise to address these issues are most useful and referral to appropriate professional care may be necessary.

8.6. Nutrition

Nutrition counselling and education on weight management are particularly important in lung disease. Up to 20–30% of normal weight individuals with COPD show a shift in body composition to muscle wasting and relative increased fat mass, independent of spirometric severity [53]. Typically, underweight status and weight loss are more prevalent in advanced disease and emphysematous phenotype [54], while obesity is more prevalent in mild disease [53]. Patients with COPD are at risk of obesity and muscle wastage due to limitations in physical activity and adverse effects of glucocorticoids given for exacerbations. For patients with COPD there is an association between underweight status and lean muscle loss and increased mortality, again independent of FEV1 [55, 56], in addition underweight patients report a lower HRQoL status then normal weight patients with COPD [57].

Changes in body weight or BMI do not accurately reflect all the changes in body composition that occur in patients with COPD. Body weight is made up of fat mass and fat free mass (FFM), fat free mass consists of water and body cell mass (organ, muscles, bone). Muscle mass constitutes a major part of fat free mass. The loss of FFM is characteristic of chronic lung diseases such as COPD and in severe COPD low FFM and mid-thigh cross sectional area have been shown to be a better predictor of prognosis than BMI [58]. Patients with COPD and low FFM have a lower exercise tolerance and impaired respiratory muscle strength than patients with maintained FFM [59–61]. FFM can be estimated using skinfold anthrometry, bioimpedance analysis or dual energy X-ray absorptiometry (DEXA).

A comprehensive pulmonary rehabilitation programme should at a minimum include a simple nutritional screening, such as calculating patient's body mass index or BMI. The aetiology of weight loss and muscle wasting in COPD is complex and a number of different physiologic and pharmacologic interventions have been used to stop or even reverse the process. This includes simple nutritional supplementation with an emphasis on adequate protein intake in order to stimulate protein synthesis to maintain or restore FFM. The increased energy requirements during activity in pulmonary rehabilitation must also be met in both underweight and normal weight individuals. Nutritional supplementation alone has not been successful in achieving significant weight gain. However, a 6 month intervention of dietary counselling along with nutritional supplementation resulted in significant weight gain and maintenance of FFM compared with control group [62].

9. Post rehabilitation assessment

9.1. Patient-centred outcomes

Patient-centred outcomes are used as outcome measures in pulmonary rehabilitation to measure the change or impact the pulmonary rehabilitation programme has had on the patient's symptoms and quality of life [6]. Outcomes used during the programme should be valid, reliable and sensitive to change and have descriptions of relevant change, such as the minimally clinical important difference, which indicate a meaningful change of the condition for better or for worse.

Outcome measures used are generally generic or disease specific, and should assess quality of life (health related quality of life, symptoms and functional impairment), depression and anxiety, functional status and breathlessness.

Exacerbation history should also be documented as an outcome measure. The same exercise test used in the pre-rehabilitation assessment (6MWT or ISWT) should also be reassessed on completion of the programme to assess for improvements in exercise capacity. Quality of life measures are used to assess symptoms, physiological functioning, functional impairment and health related quality of life [55, 63, 64]. At least one of these questionnaires is advised and may include, for example, the Chronic Respiratory Disease Questionnaire [65, 66], the St. Georges Respiratory Questionnaire [16], or the COPD Assessment Test [67]. As outlined previously, up to 40% of COPD patients have symptoms of depression and anxiety [68]. All patients should be assessed both before and after the rehabilitation programme using, for example, the Hospital Anxiety and Depression Scale [68, 69], and an onward referral to a mental health professional considered if symptoms persist significantly on completion of the programme.

Patients who are attending pulmonary rehabilitation should have the outcome of their treatment in terms of dyspnoea, health status and exercise capacity measured. Objective measurements of a patient's baseline function and post-rehabilitation function, and reassessments in the months following completion of the rehabilitation programme allows the co-ordinator to assess the benefit obtained by the individual during the programme, to provide quality assurance for the rehabilitation services and to facilitate ongoing referrals if required. Other measures of outcome, such as muscle strength, nutritional status, physical activity levels and self-efficacy measures) may also be beneficial.

10. Unanswered questions in pulmonary rehabilitation

10.1. Where is the ideal location to carry out rehabilitation?

The ideal location to carry out rehabilitation is currently unclear. The settings for pulmonary rehabilitation programmes vary; most of the research to date has involved outpatient programmes; however pulmonary rehabilitation programmes may also be conducted in an inpatient hospital or home setting. In a recent international survey involving 400 centres in 40 countries, 85% of pulmonary rehabilitation programmes in Europe and North America were using an outpatient model [70]. Outpatient settings include hospital outpatient departments, community facilities and physiotherapy clinics.

Inpatient rehabilitation is offered in hospitals and can provide specialised rehabilitation care for individuals in a stable pulmonary state or after an exacerbation. It certain cases it can be initiated during inpatient acute care including the intensive care unit where ventilator limitations may limit aerobic exercise, but resistive muscle training can be well tolerated and is associated with improved 6-minute walk distance and muscle strength [6, 71]. Potential disadvantages with inpatient rehabilitation include higher costs and lack of coverage by health insurance in certain countries.

Home based rehabilitation is an alternative model, which involves transferring the site of exercise training to the home. This could make the course more convenient and broaden the availability of the service. There is increasing evidence comparing home- and hospital-based programmes, including a recent large randomised equivalence study of home vs. outpatient rehabilitation. This demonstrated that important outcomes such as functional exercise capacity and health related quality of life were equivalent between both groups [72]. Fernandez and colleagues demonstrated that a home-based programme was safe and effective in a group of 50 patients with severe COPD on long-term supplemental oxygen [73]. There has been little uptake in clinical practice, with less than 5% of centres worldwide providing home based rehabilitation [70]. This is likely a result of limitations in some of the current studies, with many being underpowered or failing to provide all of the essential components of pulmonary rehabilitation.

The American Thoracic Society (ATS)/European Respiratory Society (ERS) Policy Statement on Pulmonary Rehabilitation identified the need to increase accessibility of pulmonary rehabilitation as a key priority, which includes investigating novel PR programme models that are more accessible and acceptable to patients [74]. Thus, when choosing a rehabilitation setting characteristics of both a particular healthcare system or setting and the patient as an individual need to be considered. Factors such as transportation, availability of various programme settings as described above and in certain countries, payment considerations and health insurance need also to be considered. In relation to patient specific factors, the severity of their disease is important, as is the haemodynamic stability of a patient often in the context of recent exacerbation, co-morbidities and extent of disability if any. These factors can influence the most appropriate setting and level of supervision a patient needs enrolling in a pulmonary rehabilitation programme.

10.2. What are the barriers to the uptake of pulmonary rehabilitation?

One key goal of pulmonary rehabilitation is ongoing lifestyle modification to encourage patients to undertake a more active lifestyle in the future. Despite the extensive evidence for its benefits, pulmonary rehabilitation is delivered to fewer than 10% with those with COPD who would benefit [52]. Accessibility is a major factor particularly in rural settings where programmes are not available or appropriate infrastructure to provide them does not exist. However, it has also been shown in metropolitan areas that up to 50% of those who are referred will never attend and of those who do present, up to a third will not complete the programme [75].

A systematic review in 2011 was carried out to identify barriers to uptake and factors affecting pulmonary rehabilitation adherence. The factors that influence whether people choose to attend their initial appointment can be different to the factors that influence programme completion [75]. A number of barriers to enrolment following referral were identified, including:

- Disruption to established routine, varying from concerns over missing social activities to work commitments or carer demands such as caring for other family members.
- Travel, transport and location, including distance to travel, available transportation or inability to travel independently.
- Influence of the referring physician – some patients declined to attend following referral by a doctor they did not know or if the perceived that their doctor did not think the rehabilitation programme would benefit them.
- Lack of perceived benefit, as some studies report patients perceiving their disease to be too severe to gain improvement or that the programme lacks guaranteed benefits.
- Inconvenient timing of the programme – patient preference on timing of rehabilitation sessions can vary between morning and afternoon, and given the limited capacity and availability not everyone's preference can be accommodated.

The definition of programme non-adherence varies in the literature from declining to participate in the programme to attending at least one session. A non-adherence rate ranging from 10 to 32% has been described and varies considerably from study to study [75]. Factors associated with non-adherence include illness and co-morbidities, travel, transportation, lack of perceived benefits, smoking, depressive symptoms and lack of support [27, 76]. Cigarette smoking at enrolment was the sole independent risk factor for non-completion of pulmonary rehabilitation, in the systematic review described above [75]. This highlights the importance of the educational component and facilitating behaviour change including programmes for strategies for smoking cessation.

10.3. How can the benefits of pulmonary rehabilitation be maintained?

Given the nature of COPD as a progressive chronic disease, it frequently results in a progressive loss of function over time. It is therefore reasonable that any benefits obtained from an initial programme are likely to regress over time [3]. The benefits of an initial pulmonary rehabilitation programme have been shown to persist to some degree for at least 12 months, with quality of life maintained better than the increased exercise capacity. Developing strategies to extend the effects of the rehabilitation programme is extremely important. The benefits of ongoing supervised maintenance exercise programmes beyond the completion of the initial cycle remains uncertain [6].

A repeat programme in those whose condition has deteriorated more than 1 year since completing the programme should be considered, and an earlier repeat programme may be warranted in those patients with a profound physiological decline within the initial 12 months of completing the programme. The benefits of a repeat programme of a patient who failed to benefit from the original programme are questionable. Ongoing exercise upon completing the programme should be encouraged in all patients, and opportunities for exercise upon completion of the programme should be provided to all patients.

Implementation of a home exercise programme at least twice a week at an early stage during the rehabilitation programme encourages the participant to exercise independently during the programme, but also improves adherence to regular exercise once the programme has been completed. Written material with an individualised description and prescription of each exercise, resembling those undertaken in the supervised classes should be provided to each participant. The programme coordinator should monitor the patients home exercise diary throughout the programme, and any barriers to exercise that the patient is experiencing should be addressed. Precautions and advice on exercise should also be addressed [20].

On completion of the programme, patients should be provided with a written, individualised, structured plan for ongoing exercise maintenance to encourage ongoing exercise. It should include aerobic and strength exercises, and information on local exercise amenities. Patients should be asked to reflect on the effect the programme has had on their daily physical activity and on their symptoms. Strategies to maintain their improvements and adherence to an ongoing exercise programme should be discussed. Regular assessments following completion of the initial programme can assist in maintaining the gains achieved during the programme [22].

10.4. Is there a role for new technology?

Pulmonary rehabilitation has rapidly established itself as a cornerstone in the comprehensive management of patients with COPD. As previously stated, a recent joint policy statement by the ATS and ERS has identified improved access and delivery of pulmonary rehabilitation to suitable patients as a priority in need of further research and development. As popularity and lack of capacity increase demand, other settings for effective rehabilitation will need to be found. These new settings would ideally maintain the quality and effectiveness of conventional programmes but be more convenient to patients [6].

New technology may play a part in improving services by telemonitoring or provision of remote rehabilitation to inaccessible regions. Telemedicine is the use of telecommunication and information technology to provide clinical health care from a distance. Telerehabilitation is the delivery of rehabilitation services over telecommunication networks and the internet, allowing point-to-point video conferencing between a central control unit and a patient at home. This is a promising way of delivering health services to individuals who may live in isolated areas without adequate access to transportation or have a level of disability which limits their ability to travel. A study carried out in 2008 used mobile phone based systems to remotely monitor an endurance exercise programme at home [77]. This programme provided a music component with an appropriate tempo to facilitate the correct intensity of training; adherence could also be monitored and appropriate feedback and support delivered. The study demonstrated good compliance and significant improvement, and was also associated with fewer exacerbations and hospitalisations [78].

There has also been evidence to support the delivery of a pulmonary rehabilitation programme from a large expert centre to smaller regional centres via videoconferencing [78]. In a controlled trial, there were equivalent outcomes for exercise capacity and quality of life. One other small trial in individuals with moderate to severe COPD, who had completed at least 12 sessions of outpatient pulmonary rehabilitation, found that telemonitoring by health care professionals reduced primary care contacts for respiratory issues compared with usual care [79]. Neither demonstrated any differences between groups and hospital admissions, days in hospital or contact with COPD nurse specialists in the community.

Education, psychosocial support and counselling are components of a pulmonary rehabilitation programme which are critical to its success. A study in 2006 demonstrated that the combination of exercise counselling, stimulation of lifestyle change or adaption and the use of a pedometer is feasible and may improve outcome and maintenance of rehabilitation results [80]. Results of a systematic review comparing home telemonitoring with usual care showed that home telehealth (home telemonitoring and telephone support) decreased rates of hospitalisation and emergency department visits, whereas findings for hospital days varied between studies. There is a great deal of variability between studies in terms of interventions and approach [81].

11. Conclusion

Pulmonary rehabilitation is one of the most cost-effective therapies for individuals with chronic respiratory disease. Despite this, many programmes are not funded adequately due to a lack of knowledge and awareness of the benefits of pulmonary rehabilitation. Healthcare professionals in clinical practice are often not familiar with the benefits, science and process of pulmonary rehabilitation, and therefore do not offer it to suitable patients. The need for standardised formal training in pulmonary rehabilitation is clear. Interestingly, even when referred, uptake of pulmonary rehabilitation by suitable patients remains poor. This may be due to a perception of pulmonary rehabilitation as being difficult or frightening. Therefore, equally important is patient education regarding the proven benefits of pulmonary rehabilitation and the processes by which those benefits are attained. Given that pulmonary rehabilitation is an evidence-based, widely-accepted gold standard treatment for many respiratory patients, the disparity in access and availability results in unacceptable inequality of healthcare [82].

Author details

Michelle Casey†, Amy Mulkerns†, Cliona O'Donnell† and Tim McDonnell*

*Address all correspondence to: timothymcdonnell@icloud.com

Department of Respiratory Medicine, St. Michaels Hospital and St. Vincent's University Hospital, Dublin, Ireland

†These authors contributed equally

References

[1] McCarthy B, et al. Pulmonary rehabilitation for chronic obstructive pulmonary disease. Cochrane Database of Systematic Reviews. 2015 Feb 23;(2):CD003793. DOI: 10.1002/14651858.CD003793.pub3

[2] Puhan M, et al. Pulmonary rehabilitation following exacerbations of chronic obstructive pulmonary disease. Cochrane Database of Systematic Reviews. 2009 Jan 21;(1):CD005305. DOI: 10.1002/14651858.CD005305.pub2

[3] Bolton CE, et al. British Thoracic Society guideline on pulmonary rehabilitation in adults. Thorax. 2013;**68**(Suppl 2):ii1-ii30

[4] Casaburi R. A brief history of pulmonary rehabilitation. Respiratory Care. 2008;**53**(9): 1185-1189

[5] Maltais F, et al. Skeletal muscle adaptation to endurancetraining in patients with chronic obstructive pulmonary disease. American Journal of Respiratory and Critical Care Medicine. 1996;**154**(2 Pt 1):442-447

[6] Spruit MA, et al. An official American Thoracic Society/European Respiratory Society statement: Key concepts and advances in pulmonary rehabilitation. American Journal of Respiratory and Critical Care Medicine. 2013;**188**(8):e13-e64

[7] Bernard S, et al. Aerobic and strength training in patients with chronic obstructive pulmonary disease. American Journal of Respiratory and Critical Care Medicine. 1999;**159**(3):896-901

[8] Griffiths TL, et al. Results at 1 year of outpatient multidisciplinary pulmonary rehabilitation: A randomised controlled trial. Lancet. 2000;**355**(9201):362-368

[9] Ries AL, et al. Effects of pulmonary rehabilitation on physiologic and psychosocial outcomes in patients with chronic obstructive pulmonary disease. Annals of Internal Medicine. 1995;**122**(11):823-832

[10] Franssen FM, et al. Effects of whole-body exercise training on body composition and functional capacity in normal-weight patients with COPD. Chest. 2004;**125**(6):2021-2028

[11] Spruit MA, et al. Resistance versus endurance training in patients with COPD and peripheral muscle weakness. The European Respiratory Journal. 2002;**19**(6):1072-1078

[12] Swallow EB, et al. Quadriceps strength predicts mortality in patients with moderate to severe chronic obstructive pulmonary disease. Thorax. 2007;**62**(2):115-120

[13] Ries AL, et al. Pulmonary rehabilitation: Joint ACCP/AACVPR evidence-based clinical practice guidelines. Chest. 2007;**131**(5 Suppl):4s-42s

[14] Casaburi R, et al. Reductions in exercise lactic acidosis and ventilation as a result of exercise training in patients with obstructive lung disease. The American Review of Respiratory Disease. 1991;**143**(1):9-18

[15] Polkey MI, Rabe KF. Chicken or egg: Physical activity in COPD revisited. European Respiratory Journal. 2009;**33**(2):227-229

[16] Jones PW, et al. A self-complete measure of health status for chronic airflow limitation: The St. George's respiratory questionnaire. American Review of Respiratory Disease. 1992;**145**(6):1321-1327

[17] Kirshner B, Guyatt G. A methodological framework for assessing health indices. Journal of Chronic Diseases. 1985;**38**(1):27-36

[18] D-C Man W, et al. Community pulmonary rehabilitation after hospitalisation for acute exacerbations of chronic obstructive pulmonary disease: Randomised controlled study. British Medical Journal. 2004;**329**(7476):1209

[19] Ries AL, et al. The effects of pulmonary rehabilitation in the national emphysema treatment trial. Chest. 2005;**128**(6):3799-3809

[20] Garvey C, et al. Pulmonary rehabilitation exercise prescription in chronic obstructive pulmonary disease: Review of selected guidelines: An official statement from The American Association of Cardiovascular and Pulmonary Rehabilitation. Journal of Cardiopulmonary Rehabilitation and Prevention. 2016;**36**(2):75-83

[21] Medicine, A.C.o.S. ACSM's Guidelines for Exercise Testing and Prescription. Philadelphia PA: Lippincott Williams & Wilkins; 2013

[22] Jenkins S, Hill K, Cecins NM. State of the art: How to set up a pulmonary rehabilitation program. Respirology. 2010;**15**(8):1157-1173

[23] Nici L, et al. American Thoracic Society/European Respiratory Society statement on pulmonary rehabilitation. American Journal of Respiratory and Critical Care Medicine. 2006;**173**(12):1390-1413

[24] Trappenburg JC, et al. Psychosocial conditions do not affect short-term outcome of multidisciplinary rehabilitation in chronic obstructive pulmonary disease. Archives of Physical Medicine and Rehabilitation. 2005;**86**(9):1788-1792

[25] Haave E, Skumlien S, Hyland ME. Gender considerations in pulmonary rehabilitation. Journal of Cardiopulmonary Rehabilitation and Prevention. 2008;**28**(3):215-219

[26] Di Meo F, et al. Age does not hamper the response to pulmonary rehabilitation of COPD patients. Age and Ageing. 2008;**37**(5):530-535

[27] Garrod R, et al. Predictors of success and failure in pulmonary rehabilitation. European Respiratory Journal. 2006;**27**(4):788

[28] Evans RA, et al. Pulmonary rehabilitation is successful for COPD irrespective of MRC dyspnoea grade. Respiratory Medicine. 2009;**103**(7):1070-1075

[29] Sabit R, et al. Predictors of poor attendance at an outpatient pulmonary rehabilitation programme. Respiratory Medicine. 2008;**102**(6):819-824

[30] Berry MJ, et al. Exercise rehabilitation and chronic obstructive pulmonary disease stage. American Journal of Respiratory and Critical Care Medicine. 1999;**160**(4):1248-1253

[31] Chavannes N, et al. Effects of physical activity in mild to moderate COPD: A systematic review. The British Journal of General Practice. 2002;**52**(480):574-578

[32] Spruit MA, et al. Effects of moderate-to-high intensity resistance training in patients with chronic heart failure. Heart. 2009;**95**(17):1399-1408

[33] Tan KH, De Cossart L, Edwards PR. Exercise training and peripheral vascular disease. The British Journal of Surgery. 2000;**87**(5):553-562

[34] Bennell KL, Hinman RS. A review of the clinical evidence for exercise in osteoarthritis of the hip and knee. Journal of Science and Medicine in Sport. 2011;**14**(1):4-9

[35] O'Gorman DJ, Krook A. Exercise and the treatment of diabetes and obesity. Medical Clinics of North America. 2011;**95**(5):953-969

[36] Rees K, et al. Exercise based rehabilitation for heart failure. Cochrane Database of Systematic Reviews. 2010 Apr 14;(4):CD003331. DOI: 10.1002/14651858.CD003331.pub3

[37] Redelmeier DA, et al. Interpreting small differences in functional status: The six minute walk test in chronic lung disease patients. American Journal of Respiratory and Critical Care Medicine. 1997;**155**(4):1278-1282

[38] Munro PE, et al. Pulmonary rehabilitation following lung transplantation. Transplantation Proceedings. 2009;**41**(1):292-295

[39] Make B. Collaborative self-management strategies for patients with respiratory disease. Respiratory Care. 1994;**39**(5):566-579 discussion 579-83

[40] Bourbeau J, Nault D, Dang-Tan T. Self-management and behaviour modification in COPD. Patient Education and Counseling. 2004;**52**(3):271-277

[41] Rice KL, et al. Disease management program for chronic obstructive pulmonary disease: A randomized controlled trial. American Journal of Respiratory and Critical Care Medicine. 2010;**182**(7):890-896

[42] Bischoff EW, et al. Effects of written action plan adherence on COPD exacerbation recovery. Thorax. 2011;**66**(1):26-31

[43] Gosselink R. Breathing techniques in patients with chronic obstructive pulmonary disease (COPD). Chronic Respiratory Disease. 2004;**1**(3):163-172

[44] Lareau S, Larson JL. Ineffective breathing pattern related to airflow limitation. The Nursing Clinics of North America. 1987;**22**(1):179-191

[45] Jones AP, Rowe BH. Bronchopulmonary hygiene physical therapy for chronic obstructive pulmonary disease and bronchiectasis. Cochrane Database of Systematic Reviews. 2000;(2):CD000045

[46] From the Global Strategy for the Diagnosis, Management and Prevention of COPD, Global Initiative for Chronic Obstructive Lung Disease (GOLD) 2017. www.goldcopd.org (cited July 2017)

[47] Spruit MA, et al. Rehabilitation and palliative care in lung fibrosis. Respirology. 2009;**14**(6):781-787

[48] Janssen DJA, et al. A call for high-quality advance care planning in outpatients with severe COPD or chronic heart failure. Chest. 2011;**139**(5):1081-1088

[49] Heffner JE. Advance care planning in chronic obstructive pulmonary disease: Barriers and opportunities. Current Opinion in Pulmonary Medicine. 2011;**17**(2):103-109

[50] Heim E, Blaser A, Waidelich E. Dyspnea: Psychophysiologic relationships. Psychosomatic Medicine. 1972;**34**(5):405-423

[51] Mills TL. Comorbid depressive symptomatology: Isolating the effects of chronic medical conditions on self-reported depressive symptoms among community-dwelling older adults. Social Science & Medicine. 2001;**53**(5):569-578

[52] Yohannes AM, Connolly MJ. Pulmonary rehabilitation programmes in the UK: A national representative survey. Clinical Rehabilitation. 2004;**18**(4):444-449

[53] Emery CF, et al. Psychological and cognitive outcomes of a randomized trial of exercise among patients with chronic obstructive pulmonary disease. Health Psychology. 1998;**17**(3):232-240

[54] Engelen MP, et al. Different patterns of chronic tissue wasting among patients with chronic obstructive pulmonary disease. Clinical Nutrition. 1999;**18**(5):275-280

[55] Schols AM, et al. Weight loss is a reversible factor in the prognosis of chronic obstructive pulmonary disease. American Journal of Respiratory and Critical Care Medicine. 1998;**157**(6 Pt 1):1791-1797

[56] Prescott E, et al. Prognostic value of weight change in chronic obstructive pulmonary disease: Results from the Copenhagen City heart study. The European Respiratory Journal. 2002;**20**(3):539-544

[57] Shoup R, et al. Body composition and health-related quality of life in patients with obstructive airways disease. European Respiratory Journal. 1997;**10**(7):1576-1580

[58] Marquis K, et al. Midthigh muscle cross-sectional area is a better predictor of mortality than body mass index in patients with chronic obstructive pulmonary disease. American Journal of Respiratory and Critical Care Medicine. 2002;**166**(6):809-813

[59] Mostert R, et al. Tissue depletion and health related quality of life in patients with chronic obstructive pulmonary disease. Respiratory Medicine. 2000;**94**(9):859-867

[60] Kobayashi A, et al. The relation of fat-free mass to maximum exercise performance in patients with chronic obstructive pulmonary disease. Lung. 2000;**178**(2):119-127

[61] Nishimura Y, et al. Relationship between respiratory muscle strength and lean body mass in men with COPD. Chest. 1995;**107**(5):1232-1236

[62] Weekes CE, Emery PW, Elia M. Dietary counselling and food fortification in stable COPD: A randomised trial. Thorax. 2009;**64**(4):326-331

[63] Taillefer M-C, et al. Health-related quality of life models: Systematic review of the literature. Social Indicators Research. 2003;**64**(2):293-323

[64] Wilson IB, Cleary PD. Linking clinical variables with health-related quality of life. A conceptual model of patient outcomes. Journal of the American Medical Association. 1995;**273**(1):59-65

[65] Guyatt GH, et al. A measure of quality of life for clinical trials in chronic lung disease. Thorax. 1987;**42**(10):773-778

[66] Williams JEA, et al. Health status measurement: Sensitivity of the self-reported chronic respiratory questionnaire (CRQ-SR) in pulmonary rehabilitation. Thorax. 2003;**58**(6):515

[67] Jones PW, et al. Development and first validation of the COPD assessment test. European Respiratory Journal. 2009;**34**(3):648

[68] Coventry PA. Does pulmonary rehabilitation reduce anxiety and depression in chronic obstructive pulmonary disease? Current Opinion in Pulmonary Medicine. 2009;**15**(2): 143-149

[69] Zigmond AS, Snaith RP. The hospital anxiety and depression scale. Acta Psychiatrica Scandinavica. 1983;**67**(6):361-370

[70] Spruit MA, et al. Differences in content and organisational aspects of pulmonary rehabilitation programmes. European Respiratory Journal. 2014;**43**(5):1326-1337

[71] Troosters T, et al. Resistance training prevents deterioration in quadriceps muscle function during acute exacerbations of chronic obstructive pulmonary disease. American Journal of Respiratory and Critical Care Medicine. 2010;**181**(10):1072-1077

[72] Holland AE, et al. Home-based rehabilitation for COPD using minimal resources: A randomised, controlled equivalence trial. Thorax. 2016

[73] Fernandez AM, et al. Home-based pulmonary rehabilitation in very severe COPD: Is it safe and useful? Journal of Cardiopulmonary Rehabilitation and Prevention. 2009;**29**(5):325-331

[74] Rochester CL. An official American Thoracic Society/European Respiratory Society policy statement: Enhancing implementation, use, and delivery of pulmonary rehabilitation. Am J Respir Crit Care Med. 2015;**192**(11):1373-1386

[75] Keating A, Lee A, Holland AE. What prevents people with chronic obstructive pulmonary disease from attending pulmonary rehabilitation? A systematic review. Chronic Respiratory Disease. 2011;**8**(2):89-99

[76] Hogg L, et al. Effectiveness, attendance, and completion of an integrated, system-wide pulmonary rehabilitation service for COPD: Prospective observational study. Chronic Obstructive Pulmonary Disease. 2012;**9**(5):546-554

[77] Liu WT, et al. Efficacy of a cell phone-based exercise programme for COPD. The European Respiratory Journal. 2008;**32**(3):651-659

[78] Stickland M, et al. Using Telehealth technology to deliver pulmonary rehabilitation in chronic obstructive pulmonary disease patients. Canadian Respiratory Journal. 2011;**18**(4):216-220

[79] Lewis KE, et al. Does home telemonitoring after pulmonary rehabilitation reduce healthcare use in optimized COPD? A pilot randomized trial. Chronic Obstructive Pulmonary Disease. 2010;**7**(1):44-50

[80] de Blok BM, et al. The effects of a lifestyle physical activity counseling program with feedback of a pedometer during pulmonary rehabilitation in patients with COPD: A pilot study. Patient Education and Counseling. 2006;**61**(1):48-55

[81] Polisena J, et al. Home telehealth for chronic obstructive pulmonary disease: A systematic review and meta-analysis. Journal of Telemedicine and Telecare. 2010;**16**(3):120-127

[82] Vogiatzis I, et al. American Journal of Respiratory and Critical Care Medicine

Chapter 7

Advances in Pulmonary Rehabilitation for Chronic Obstructive Pulmonary Disease and Associated Conditions

Ipek Candemir

Additional information is available at the end of the chapter

http://dx.doi.org/10.5772/intechopen.70920

Abstract

Pulmonary rehabilitation (PR) is an evidenced-based, proven treatment as mentioned recent guidelines in patients with chronic obstructive pulmonary disease (COPD). Exercise training is a cornerstone of PR programs, Inspiratory muscle training, neuromuscular electrical stimulation (NMES) are effective in selected patients. Water-based rehabilitation and tai chi are well tolerated recent modalities. Although there is an absence of a specific PR protocol for special conditions, PR is recommended before and also after endobronchial volume reduction (EBVR), lung volume reduction surgery (LVRS), both before and after lung transplantation periods, before, after surgery, during the intensive care unit (ICU) period, the chemotherapy period and as a component of palliative care. After COPD exacerbation, it is recommended within 3 weeks of hospital discharge. Modifying PR programs while considering comorbidities might lead to greater improvement in outcomes. After PR, the important points are to follow prescribed home exercise programs, control programs in the PR center/unit, and being more active in daily living life for the purpose of preserving improvements. Tele-PR is an alternative to conventional modalities due to similar improvements. Although PR is effective, it is an underutilized resource. The awareness of PR should be increased in patients and among health professionals.

Keywords: PR, exercise capacity, quality of life, perioperative lung transplantation, EBVR

1. Introduction

Chronic obstructive pulmonary disease (COPD), a systemic progressive disease that results in reduced exercise capacity and quality of life, progressive dyspnea, and mortality. It causes health and economic burdens unless pharmacologic and nonpharmacologic treatments are optimized. One of the most important interventions is pulmonary rehabilitation (PR). It is a proven modality and is included in COPD treatment guidelines. The evidence-based benefits are improvement in exercise capacity and quality of life, recovery time after hospitalization, and survival; and reduction in perceived intensity of breathlessness, number of hospitalizations, and days in hospital; and enhancement of the effect of long-acting bronchodilators. Although most studies included patients with moderate-to-severe COPD and demonstrated evidence for these patients, PR is recommended for all patients who are symptomatic with reduced exercise capacity and quality of life, regardless of disease severity. PR is also an effective, feasible modality during the intensive care unit (ICU) period and early periods after exacerbation. The recommended time for PR is during the perioperative period in lung transplantation. Additionally, PR is required before endobronchial volume reduction (EBVR) and has shown to be beneficial before and after lung cancer surgery. This chapter outlines the pathophysiologies that give rise to indications for PR, the latest developments in PR, and PR modalities associated with COPD.

2. The definition of PR

PR is described as "a comprehensive intervention based on a thorough patient assessment followed by patient-tailored therapies that include, but are not limited to, exercise training, education, and behavior changes, that is designed to improve the physical and psychological conditions of people with chronic respiratory disease, and to promote the long-term adherence to health-enhancing behaviors [1]."

3. Pathophysiologies indicated for PR

3.1. Exercise limitation

Exercise intolarence is one of the most important and common symptoms experienced by patients with mild-to-severe COPD and are related to reduced health-related quality of life. Exercise intolerance in patients with COPD is primarily due to impaired ventilatory mechanics, but it is also associated with gas exchange limitation, cardiovascular factors, peripheral skeletal muscle dysfunction and a combination of these [2, 3]. Additionally, anxiety and poor motivation are other factors of exercise intolerance. Although the exact association has yet to be found, it is thought that anxiety and depression contribute to exercise intolerance [4], due to the effect that these have on increased symptom perception [5, 6].

Ventilatory limitation: Multiple factors determine ventilatory limitation, which consists of abnormalities in ventilatory mechanics and ventilatory muscle function. Other reasons for ventilatory limitation are increased ventilatory demands as a result of changes in gas exchange, and discordance in the neuroregulatory control of breathing. The most important pathophysiology in patients with COPD is expiratory flow limitation. During exercise, air becomes trapped, which results in dynamic lung hyperinflation (DH) above the already increased resting volumes. Additionally, DH inhibits tidal volume expansion during exercise and contributes to cardiac dysfunction by increasing the positive intrathoracic pressures, which likely contribute to cardiac impairment [7].

Gas exchange limitation: Hypoxia is likely to limit exercise tolerance. Hypoxia increases pulmonary ventilation by enhancing output of peripheral chemoreceptors and production of lactic acid. Lactic acidemia results in increased pulmonary ventilation because of an increase in carbon dioxide production due to buffered lactic acid [8]. Above the lactic threshold, severe dyspnea correlates with increased work rates. Dyspnea may quickly increase. Furthermore, plasma norepinephrine and epinephrine also increase during exercise [9, 10].

Cardiovascular factors: In patients with COPD, the cardiovascular system is influenced by various mechanisms. The most important is an increase in right ventricular afterload through elevated pulmonary vascular resistance from direct vascular injury [11, 12], hypoxic vasoconstriction [13], and/or increases in effective pulmonary vascular resistance due to erythrocytosis [14]. In the course of time, the overloaded right ventricle leads to right ventricular hypertrophy, which could result in right ventricular failure [15]. During exercise, pulmonary vascular resistance is rapidly increased due to breathing at lung volumes close to total lung capacity [16, 17]. Lung hyperinflation and excessive expiratory muscle recruitment are likely to reduce venous return and right ventricular preload in COPD [18, 19]. Moreover, during exercise, large intrathoracic pressure swings for the purpose of overcoming the increased elastic and resistive loads, may result in left ventricular dysfunction by increasing left ventricular afterload [20, 21]. These right ventricular effects can also compromise left ventricular filling through septal shifts that further reduce the ability of the heart to meet exercise demands [22].

Peripheral skeletal muscle dysfunction: Skeletal muscle dysfunction in patients with COPD is characterized by remarkably decreased muscle strength and endurance. The mechanisms are reduction in muscle mass and proportion of oxidative fibers, increases in the proportion of glycolytic fibers and muscle atrophy, and also a detoriation of oxidative metabolic capacity due to reductions in mitochondrial enzyme activities and capillary density. Additionally, systemic inflammation; malnutrition; corticosteroid use; hypoxemia; aging; smoking; the production of reactive oxygen and nitrogen species; enhanced protein degradation inside muscle fibers; increased activities of the proteasomal and lysosomal pathways; and activation of calpains and caspases contribute to muscle dysfunction. Therefore, patients with COPD enter into a vicious circle owing to disuse and inactivity due to the aforementioned mechanisms [23].

3.2. Body composition disorders

Unexplained weight loss occurs in about 50% of patients with severe COPD and 15% of patients with mild-to-moderate COPD [24, 25]. The main cause of weight loss in COPD is the reduction in skeletal muscle mass rather than loss of fat mass. Based on the reduction of fat mass or fat-free mass index (FFMI), nutritional abnormalities in COPD have been categorized into four types. Normal body mass index (BMI) with normal FFMI is normal, low BMI with normal or above-normal FFMI is defined as semistarvation, normal or above-normal BMI with low FFMI is defined as muscle atrophy, and low BMI with low FFMI as cachexia [26]. There are several reasons for weight loss in patients with COPD, even if during a stable period. In patients with stable COPD, there is an increased metabolic rate due to abnormal respiratory dynamics, chronic systemic inflammation, and drugs [27–31]. In malnourished mobile patients with COPD, although the basal metabolic rate is reduced, the resting energy expenditure is high. During exercise, inefficient muscle contractions due to increased consumption of adenosine triphosphate are added on. Also, there is an increase in the levels of inflammatory cytokines such as tumor necrosis factor-alpha (TNF-α) and interleukin (IL) 1 in circulation. TNF-α and IL1 have been shown to contribute to weight loss even in healthy individuals [32].

3.3. Psychological status

Patients with COPD have a higher prevalence of depression and anxiety than the general population [33] and a higher risk for developing depression [34]. The etiology of the association between depression and COPD has not been revealed clearly. The most important risk factor for COPD is smoking. Depressed individuals are more likely to smoke [35], have a tendency to smoking [36, 37], and find smoking cessation more difficult [35, 38]. Conversely, smokers are more likely to be depressed [39], which could be caused by activation of nicotinic acetylcholine receptors [40], and the inflammatory effects of smoking [41]. Soluble tumor necrosis factor receptor-1 has shown to be associated with rates of depression in patients with COPD [42], but there is not exact relationship between TNF-α and COPD [43, 44]. Hypoxia is thought be an additional factor in the development of depression in COPD. Low arterial oxygen saturation has been shown to be associated with periventricular white matter lesions [45], which are found in patients with depression [46]. Other important risk factors are the severity of symptoms and reported quality of life [47]. Depression is found more frequently in support-bound patients with COPD [48].

4. Content of PR programs

4.1. Exercise training

Exercise training is a cornerstone of PR programs. Exercise training is shown to be the best approach for increasing muscle strength, is likely to improve motivation for exercise, reduce mood abnormalities [49, 50], decrease symptoms [51], and improve cardiovascular function [1]. As recent major guidelines recommend, the main components of exercise training programs for patients with COPD are endurance and resistance training, which should be included in PR programs. Although none of the guidelines make clear, specific, and accurate recommendations for whole exercise training, they agree on endurance training at least 3 to 5 times weekly >60% of the maximal work rate. However, there is no consensus of initial workloads or in increasing the exercise load or program duration; the duration of exercise is recommended for at least 20 minutes and a target program duration of up to 12 weeks [52].

Inspiratory muscle training (IMT): Respiratory muscle training is a part of rehabilitation in selected patients with COPD. Respiratory strength has been found to correlate with improved pulmonary function, reduction of dyspnea severity, improved exercise tolerance, and enhanced functionality and quality of life [53, 54]. IMT is thought to contribute to contraction of the diaphragm by increasing type II fibers [55], which results in reduced inspiratory time [56] and subsequently increased expiratory time. Hyperinflation is expected to eventually diminish [57]; therefore, IMT is thought to impact on dyspnea without any significant change in inspiratory pressure [58, 59].

Neuromuscular electrical stimulation (NMES): NMES is one of the recent rehabilitation modalities that involve passive stimulation of contraction of the peripheral muscles through the application of an electric current via electrodes placed on the skin over the targeted muscles by depolarizing motor neurons. It aims to elicit beneficial training effects without causing dyspnea in patients who are unable to participate in PR programs. The stimulation-pulse duration is usually 250–400 μs, and stimulation frequency ranges from 8 to 120 Hz. Intensities range from 10 to 100 mA, and these are gradually increased throughout the entire stimulation according to the patient's individual tolerance. In a meta-analysis published in 2016, it was found that NMES improved quadriceps strength and exercise capacity; however, there was no statistically significant improvement in the degree of health-related quality of life in patients with moderate-to-severe COPD [60]. In several studies, it has been reported that NMES had an impact on the increase in type II fiber cross-sectional area with a decrease in type I fiber cross-sectional area of the muscle, and on the decrease in muscle oxidative stress in patients with COPD. Owing to the fact that NMES has a low impact on ventilation, heart rate, and dyspnea, it could be applied during periods of exacerbation, and during admission to the ICU for acute COPD exacerbation [61, 62].

Recent exercise training approaches: Besides conventional exercise trainings, there have been a few papers published recently about alternative exercise training modalities in patients with COPD. According to these studies, water-based rehabilitation [63] and tai chi were found as well tolerated and enjoyable [64, 65].

4.2. Other interventions

PR programs should be comprehensive and individualized according to patients' needs. Other interventions are breathing strategies, bronchial hygiene techniques, psychological and nutritional recommendations and support if needed, and education of patients and care givers. Body composition abnormalities, especially malnutrition, have already been found to increase risks of mortality among patients with COPD. A significant improvement has been shown in pulmonary function in patients with COPD who have a higher fat, lower carbohydrate diet than the traditional high-carbohydrate diet [66]. Omega-3 polyunsaturated fatty acids (PUFA) have been shown to have an antiinflammatory effect and be effective in patients with COPD [67]. It is also important to relapse any deficiency of vitamin D due to the association with early progression, myopathy/muscle weakness, and the immune-modulatory effect of vitamin D [27].

5. Outcomes and response to PR

It has been demonstrated that PR is the most effective therapeutic approach for improving dyspnea, health status, and exercise tolerance [68]. It is also one of the most cost effective therapeutic strategies. Additionally, it reduces hospitalizations among patients who have had recent exacerbations [69]. Improvements are seen among all grades of COPD severity, but recommendations are stronger in moderate-to-severe COPD. In some studies, improvements of outcomes were seen regardless of baseline lung function, dyspnea, and exercise capacity [70].

5.1. Exercise capacity

Various exercise tests are used for evaluating exercise capacity, the mechanisms of main disruption, and the response to PR. Some are also strong independent prognostic factors in patients with COPD. There are several laboratory-based exercise tests that use either maximal incremental or constant workload protocols to evaluate exercise performance after PR. Field tests are more widely used and more practical to perform. The six-minute walk test (6MWT), incremental and endurance shuttle walk test (ISWT, ESWT) are standardized and have also been used in PR and various clinical trials. In COPD, endurance tests [constant work rate exercise test (CWRET) and ESWT] are more responsive to interventions than other types of tests. The cycle ergometer CWRET has been used more widely than ESWT. By using CWRET, the work rate, inspiratory capacity, and isotime responses, which verify potential mechanisms of improvement or deterioration, are accurately measured [71].

The ISWT is a significant predictor of survival, readmission, and is usually sensitive to PR in patients with COPD [72]. In a recent meta-analysis of nine trials, a mean improvement of 38 m was found [68]. After recovering from a stay in the ICU, ISWT was found to improve by a mean of 64 m after rehabilitation [72]. ESWT duration was found as moderately correlated with FEV1, but not with muscle mass or strength in patients with COPD [73]. ESWT is responsive to PR improving by 100–400 s. [71]. According to a meta-analysis of rehabilitative interventions in COPD, the mean effect of rehabilitation on 6MWD was 44 m when treatment and control groups were compared [74].

Peak oxygen uptake (V′O2peak) shows the highest oxygen uptake during incremental exercise tests by achieving the subject's limit of tolerance. With good subject effort, V′O2peak is closely reflective of the subject's "maximum" V′O2, the gold standard index of aerobic capacity [75]. There is very little information about what constitutes a minimal clinically important difference (MCID) in V′O2peak. In the National Emphysema Treatment Trial (NETT), 4 ± 1 W was considered the symptoms-anchored MCID in patients with severe COPD [76], with a V′O2peak change of $\sim 0.04 \pm 0.01$ $L{\cdot}min^{-1}$. In several studies including patients with Global Initiative for Chronic Obstructive Lung Disease (GOLD) stages 2–4 COPD V′O2peak has been shown to moderately significantly increase after lower limb endurance muscle training. After PR in patients with COPD, V′O2peak was found to be in the range 0.1–0.5 $L{\cdot}min^{-1}$ or ~10–40% of baseline, with a mean improvement of ~11% [77, 78].

5.2. Health-related quality of life daily living activities

In a recent study, it was aimed to determine the responsiveness of St. George's Respiratory Questionnaire (SGRQ), COPD Assessment Test (CAT), COPD Clinical Questionnaire (CCQ), and Hospital Anxiety and Depression Scale (HADS) to PR in 419 patients with COPD, and also estimate the MCID for CAT, CCQ, and HADS. It was demonstrated that SGRQ, CAT,

CCQ, and HADS were responsive to PR in patients with moderate-to-very-severe COPD. The calculated MCID ranges were −3.0 to −2.0 points for CAT; −0.5 to −0.3 points for CCQ; −1.8 to −1.3 points for HADS-A, and −1.7 to −1.5 points for HADS-D [79].

6. PR in special conditions

6.1. Before and after transplantation

Lung transplantation is a recommended intervention in patients with advanced-stage pulmonary disease who are unresponsive to pharmacologic and nonpharmacologic treatment. Factors such as chronic respiratory failure, cardiovascular risk factors, muscular and nutritional conditions, which are likely to influence the prognosis for a successful lung transplantation, usually accompany advanced chronic respiratory disorders. Therefore, PR is an important approach that modifies and controls potential risk factors. PR plays an important role for the maintenance of exercise tolerance and physical functioning [80] both before and after the lung transplantation because common extra pulmonary manifestations could be persistent or deteriorate. As such, PR is recommended both before and after lung transplantation. Although there is an absence of a specific PR protocol for patients for lung transplant, it was shown to improve maximal and functional exercise capacity, quality of life, and skeletal muscle function [81].

Before transplantation: The role of PR in preoperative patients is essential for quitting smoking, improving body composition, optimizing medical treatment, and restoring patients' independence for functioning, relieving symptoms, decreasing disability, and improving quality of life by increasing their participation in social and physical activities. It has been shown that the rate of success in lung transplantation was linked to exercise capacity and resting carbon dioxide in arterial blood values [82]. Those parameters were also found to predict hospital stay after surgery and mortality. Additionally, pretransplant PR was also found to be associated with decreased posttransplant ICU days, mechanical ventilation, and chest tube days and survey [83]. Multidisciplinary, comprehensive PR must be individualized and the modality and intensity of training must be selected for each patient. The duration of training can vary from 6 weeks to 6 months [84]. The program should consist of education (including the following topics: bronchial hygiene, breathing control techniques, relaxation, education about COPD, and education of relatives and energy conservation), exercise training (upper and lower limb aerobic exercise, resistance training, flexibility, inspiratory muscle training), psychological support, and nutritional support. The intensity of exercise is dynamically increased according to the progress of each individual patient.

After transplantation: Although pulmonary functions are improved after transplantation, limited exercise capacity is persistent due to different mechanisms. Persistent limited exercise capacity is not only associated with ventilatory or cardiovascular factors [85, 86], skeletal muscle dysfunction is the main problem. Skeletal muscle changes include impaired oxidative capacity, lactate threshold changes, and a lower proportion of type I muscle fibers [87]. A sedentary life style both before and after transplantation contributes to skeletal muscle weakness [88]. Hospitalizations due to infections or acute rejections and the use of immunosuppressive medication further impact muscle function in lung recipients [89]. It was found that V′O2 peak was 45–52% predicted in patients after lung transplantation for up to 2 years. Patients stop exercise because of leg fatigue, rather than dyspnea [90]. Additionally, maximal cycle-work capacity correlates better with isokinetic cycling work capacity than with pulmonary function after lung transplantation [91]. PR should be started in the ICU with positioning of the patient, ventilation of all lung lobes, and mobilization of secretions by managing cough. Deep breathing exercises should be initiated because tachypnoea and pursed-lip breathing persist postoperatively and old breathing patterns must be overcome. Sitting and mobilization out of bed should then be performed. After all chest drains have been removed, walking or cycle ergometry should performed. Muscle strength and function, and endurance training should focus on lower extremities, and weights can be limited to 3 kg initially for upper extremities [92]. After discharge, patients should be referred to PR center/units as soon as possible. Although there is no consensus on optimal exercise training and education programs, aerobic and strength exercise training of the lower and upper extremities 2–3 times per week for 6–8 weeks, are recommended. The intensity of exercise can be increased according to patient tolerance. High-intensity aerobic exercise training at 60–80% of maximal work capacity has been found to be correlated with physiologic improvements in patients with stable COPD. Hence, high-intensity training is preferred. Interval training could be applied in patients who cannot sustain continuous high-intensity. Stretching, flexibility, and chest-mobility exercises may also be an important component of exercise after LVRS or transplantation [1, 82, 93]. Education of patients and care givers is also an important issue.

6.2. Lung volume resection surgery (LVRS)

Similar recommendations are valid for LVRS, which is not usually an effective intervention for exercise intolerance and functional disability. Baseline skeletal muscle dysfunction, time needed to achieve postoperative improvement in lung function (peak benefits are usually seen 6–12 months after surgery), and inactivity/immobility associated with the perioperative period are factors that reduce exercise capacity. Several studies compared the benefits of LVRS and several-weeks'–duration comprehensive PR in patients with severe emphysema. PR was found to significantly improve exercise tolerance, health status, and dyspnea, without significant changes in lung function as compared with PR and LVRS, even if highly selected patients showed significantly better improvement in lung function [94–97], exercise capacity [95–97], and quality of life [96, 97].

6.3. Endobronchial volume reduction (EBVR)

Endobronchial volume reduction interventions result in improved spirometric measures and 6MWD at 6 months, only if in correctly selected subjects. PR is recommended before and after EBVR, which is indicated in the presence of persistent dyspnea despite maximal medical therapy and PR, and reduced exercise capacity (6MWD ≥140 m after rehabilitation) [97].

6.4. Lung cancer

In patients with lung cancer, exercise limitations can be due to the effects of the cancer, coexisting morbidities, and/or the effects of treatment and surgery. Cancer-related anemia, and muscle atrophy and dysfunction contribute to limited exercise capacity. Inactivity due to cancer and its comorbidities further compound this situation. In the pre- and postoperative period, quitting smoking, optimizing COPD medical treatment, educating patients, prophylaxis for thrombosis, and PR are the recommended approaches that decrease risks. PR is an effective and feasible intervention before and after surgery, during the chemotherapy period, and as a component of palliative care. Even though PR consists of an exercise program for lower and upper extremities, breathing, airway clearance techniques, oxygen therapy, bronchodilator optimization, and self-management training similar to other conditions, it should also be individualized and multidisciplinary in patients with cancer.

Even though surgical procedures have improved and patients are highly selected, morbidity and mortality rates are still increasing as a consequence of cardiopulmonary complications after surgery. Limited exercise capacity as a modifiable risk factor is the best independent predictor of postoperative complications. Multidisciplinary preoperative PR improves exercise capacity and postoperative recovery, and reduces hospital stay and pulmonary infections [98]. During the chemotherapy period, symptoms such as fatigue, breathlessness, and quality of life are likely to deteriorate. Exercise training improves fatigue, aerobic capacity, muscular strength, and physical and functional activity in patients with cancer, even though they are undergoing chemotherapy [99]. Breathing techniques and medications that result in reduced inflammation and opened airways in combination with exercise training have recently become a part of supportive care for patients undergoing chemotherapy and radiation therapy [100]. PR plays a role in the management of terminal cancer. Exercise training modalities include walking with/without assistance or device, passive or active strengthening exercises, continuous passive motion, passive or active range of motion, NMES, and pain management interventions such as massage and heating pads [101]. Oxygen therapy has an important role in palliative care because it both treats hypoxemia and reduces the sensation of dyspnea. Additionally, education about mobilization with assistive devices, environmental modification, energy conservation, and work simplification techniques are also beneficial. These interventions have been investigated and were shown to be effective in cancer-related fatigue in several studies [102–104]. In another study, it was shown that exercise training decreased anxiety, stress, depression, and there were improvements in pain, fatigue, shortness of breath, constipation, and insomnia in patients with cancer, even at advanced stages [105].

6.5. Exacerbation of COPD

COPD exacerbations are known to deteriorate life quality, disease progression, and mortality. The British Thoracic Society (BTS) recommends the initiation of PR within 1 month of hospital discharge after exacerbation, consisting of a minimum of twice-weekly supervised sessions lasting between 6 and 12 weeks [106]. Exercise should combine progressive muscle resistance and aerobic training [106]. Systematic reviews have shown that quality of life and daily functioning were improved with large and important clinical effects of PR [107, 108]. According to the European Respiratory Society (ERS)/American Thoracic Society (ATS) guidelines of management of COPD exacerbations, PR added to medical treatment during hospitalization increases mortality [109]; however, NMES and resisted quadriceps exercises performed during hospitalization during exacerbation have been shown to improve muscle strength without increasing systemic inflammation. PR that is started within 3 weeks of discharge following a COPD exacerbation reduces hospital admissions, improves quality of life, and also increases exercise capacity when implemented within 8 weeks of discharge. Although the best approach is indistinct and further investigations are necessary, a combination of regular exercise with breathing technique training has been shown to be superior [109].

6.6. PR in the intensive unit care

In the ICU, skeletal muscle mass is lost at a rate of 5% per week. This neuromuscular weakness has been found to be correlated with the duration of mechanical ventilation, and associated with functional disability and decreased quality of life for up to 5 years after hospitalization. Mobilization and rehabilitation of critically ill patients might improve physical functioning and decrease duration of mechanical ventilation and ICU length of stay [110, 111]. A meta-analysis was published in 2017 that consisted of studies with PR programs containing patient mobilization, walking, standing, breathing exercises, in-bed supine cycle ergometry, passive-active range of motion (ROM), and NMES. It was shown that early mobilization and physical rehabilitation of critically ill patients seemed to be safe, with a low risk of potential safety events, even if as a usual care. Although the definition of safety assessments was heterogeneous, it was emphasized that the awareness and implementation of existing recommendations should be increased [112].

6.7. Patients with hypercapnia

Hypercapnia is an indicator of alveolar hypoventilation due to an overload on the ventilatory pump that is greater than its capacity. In patients with COPD, diminished ventilatory response usually results in chronic retention of carbon dioxide. Chronic respiratory failure is frequently seen in the end stage of the progression of COPD. In the BTS guidelines, it is mentioned that patients with chronic respiratory failure gain as much benefit as those without chronic respiratory failure from PR with level 3 evidence [106]. A study showed that pCO2 levels were significantly more reduced in patients with COPD with pursed-lip and diaphragmatic breathing exercises during hospitalization period than in a control group. It was suggested that respiratory exercise training was quite effective in reducing pCO2 levels. As the guidelines recommend, patients with COPD should be referred for PR regardless of having chronic respiratory failure [113].

Noninvasive mechanical ventilation (NIMV): Noninvasive mechanical ventilation (NIMV) reduces breathlessness and increases exercise tolerance by reducing the acute load on the respiratory muscles. According to these mechanisms, the effect of NIMV on PR outcomes has been investigated in several studies in which NIMV was applied during exercise training or at night. In a review of the Cochrane Database in which the effect of NIMV was investigated during exercise training as a part of PR, it was shown that NIMV during exercise training improved exercise capacity of the lower limbs, and enabled exercise at higher training intensities. There was no definite evidence about quality of life and none of the studies investigated the effect of NIMV during exercise training on physical activity [114]. It has also been shown that exercise tolerance and quality of life were improved in patients with severe COPD using nocturnal NIMV after PR, presumably through resting the respiratory muscles at night [115]. As a recommendation of the ERS/ATS guidelines, NIMV could be an adjunctive therapy to unload the respiratory muscles for the purpose of increasing the intensity of exercise training in selected patients with severe chronic respiratory disease who have a suboptimal response to exercise [1].

6.8. Comorbidities

The most common comorbidities associated with COPD are cardiovascular disease, orthopedic problems, metabolic disease, depression, and anxiety. It is expected that comorbidities may effect the outcomes of PR as an impact on COPD outcomes such as quality of life, health care costs, and mortality rate. Various comorbidities such as anxiety and depression, cardiovascular disease, metabolic disease, and osteoporosis affected PR outcomes in some studies [116–121]; a meta-analysis could not be performed according to the heterogeneous results. Only four studies investigated the influence of the number of comorbidities on PR outcomes. Three of which showed that the number of comorbidities was not related to PR outcomes [117, 119, 120]. A study showed that metabolic disease negatively influenced 6MWT distance, whereas cardiac disease negatively influenced the St. George's Respiratory Questionnaire [118]. A prior study of patients with COPD with osteoarthritis and neurologic problems who were assigned to water-based exercise training reported a greater improvement in outcomes compared with land-based exercise training [121]. Previous studies have identified that patients with psychiatric problems experienced a lesser improvement in dyspnea [117], and patients with metabolic disease demonstrated a greater improvement in dyspnea after PR compared with controls [118]. A study was published in 2017 that included 165 patients with COPD with exercise limitations. Comorbidity was classified as cardiac, metabolic, orthopedic, behavioral health problems, or other diseases. Comorbidities were found to have no effect on the maximal incremental exercise test and constant workload cycle endurance time after PR. Patients with cardiac disease were found to have greater improvements in dyspnea scores than those with no cardiac disease, and patients with orthopedic problems had a smaller but clinically significant improvement in dyspnea after PR [122]. Modifying PR programs with consideration to comorbidities might lead to greater improvement in outcomes, but how to structure programs according to comorbidities is still to be determined.

7. Follow-up programs of PR and Tele-PR

The best and the most effective follow-up program have not been found. After PR, the important points are to follow prescribed home exercise programs and follow-up programs in the PR center/unit, and to be more active in daily living life for the purpose of preserving improvements. Accordingly, family members have a role that is as important as that of the PR center staff in encouraging and motivating the patients. In a cohort of patients with COPD who completed a 10-week comprehensive PR program, a structured follow-up home program was prescribed and the patients were monitored for 1 year. At the 1-year follow-up evaluation, only the patients who continued with the home program had maintained the improvements of the initial PR program in endurance capacity, and psychological and cognitive functioning [123, 124]. Despite the clear benefits of PR, it is often an under-utilized resource. Limited access and poor adherence result in <5% of eligible people with COPD receiving PR each year. Although the traditional models of inpatient and outpatient PR are suitable for many patients, alternative models may also be effective and may improve patient access, particularly in regions or healthcare systems where traditional models of PR are not feasible. For example, tele-rehabilitation, which links expert rehabilitation healthcare providers with others at a remote site or with patients in their homes, also has the potential to improve access [125]. A recent study showed that home-based maintenance tele-rehabilitation was equally as effective as hospital-based, outpatient, maintenance PR in reducing the risk for acute exacerbations of COPD and hospitalizations with lower risk for emergency department visits. It was suggested that tele-rehabilitation was likely to be an effective alternative strategy to hospital-based, outpatient, maintenance PR. In addition, it had a potential economic advantage compared with standard PR [126]. Tele-PR has been developed to improve patients' participation and treatment adherence, but the most important point is awareness. The awareness of PR should be increased in patients and among health professionals.

Author details

Ipek Candemir

Address all correspondence to: ipekcayli@yahoo.com

Ataturk Chest Disease and Chest Surgery Research and Education Hospital, Ankara, Turkey

References

[1] Spruit MA, Singh SJ, Garvey C, ZuWallack R, Nici L, Rochester C, et al. An official American Thoracic Society/European Respiratory Society statement: Key concepts and advances in pulmonary rehabilitation. American Journal of Respiratory and Critical Care Medicine. 2013;**188**(8):13-64

[2] MacIntyre NR. Mechanisms of functional loss in patients with chronic lung disease. Respiratory Care. 2008;**53**(9):1177-1184

[3] European Respiratory Society Task Force. Clinical exercise testing with reference to lung diseases: Indications, standardization and interpretation strategies. The European Respiratory Journal. 1997;**10**(11):2662-2689

[4] Borak J, Chodosowska E, Matuszewski A, Zielinski J. Emotional status does not alter exercise tolerance in patients with chronic obstructive pulmonary disease. The European Respiratory Journal. 1998;**12**:370-373

[5] Janson C, Bjornsson E, Hetta J, Boman G. Anxiety and depression in relation to respiratory symptoms and asthma. American Journal of Respiratory and Critical Care Medicine. 1994;**149**:930-934

[6] Parekh PI, Blumenthal JA, Babyak MA, Merrill K, Carney RM, Davis RD, Palmer SM. Psychiatric disorder and quality of life in patients awaiting lung transplantation. Chest. 2003;**124**:1682-1688

[7] O'Donnell DE. Ventilatory limitations in chronic obstructive pulmonary disease. Medicine and Science in Sports and Exercise. 2001 Jul;**33**(7 Suppl):S647-S655

[8] Somfay A, Porszasz J, Lee SM, Casaburi R. Effect of hyperoxia on gas exchange and lactate kinetics following exercise onset in nonhypoxemic COPD patients. Chest. 2002;**121**:393-400

[9] Wasserman K, Hansen JE, Sue DY, Stringer W, Whipp BJ. Principles of Exercise Testing and Interpretation. 4th ed. Philadelphia: Lippincott Williams & Wilkins; 2005. p. 41

[10] Weltman A, Wood CM, Womack CJ, Davis SE, Blumer JL, Alvarez J, et al. Catecholamine and blood lactate responses to incremental rowing and running exercise. Journal of Applied Physiology. 1994;**76**(3):1144-1149

[11] World Health Organization. Definition of chronic corpulmonale. Circulation. 1963;**27**: 594-615

[12] Santos S, Peinado VI, Ramirez J, Melgosa T, Roca J, Rodriguez-Roisin R, Barbera JA. Characterization of pulmonary vascular remodelling in smokers and patients with mild COPD. The European Respiratory Journal. 2002;**19**:632-638

[13] Voelkel NF, Tuder RM. Hypoxia-induced pulmonary vascular remodeling: A model for what human disease? The Journal of Clinical Investigation. 2000;**106**:733-738

[14] Chetty KG, Brown SE, Light RW. Improved exercise tolerance of the polycythemic lung patient following phlebotomy. The American Journal of Medicine. 1983;**74**:415-420

[15] Sietsema K. Cardiovascular limitations in chronic pulmonary disease. Medicine and Science in Sports and Exercise. 2001;**33**:S656-S661

[16] Ranieri VM, Dambrosio M, Brienza N. Intrinsic PEEP and cardiopulmonary interaction in patients with COPD and acute ventilatory failure. The European Respiratory Journal. 1996;**9**:1283-1292

[17] Oswald-Mammosser M, Kessler R, Massard G, et al. Effect of lung volume reduction surgery on gas exchange and pulmonary hemodynamics at rest and during exercise. American Journal of Respiratory and Critical Care Medicine. 1998;**158**:1020-1025

[18] Mahler DA, Brent BN, Loke J, et al. Right ventricular performance and central circulatory hemodynamics during upright exercise in patients with chronic obstructive pulmonary disease. The American Review of Respiratory Disease. 1984;**130**:722-729

[19] Miller JD, Pegelow DF, Jacques AJ, et al. Effects of augmented respiratory muscle pressure production on locomotor limb venous return during calf contraction exercise. Journal of Applied Physiology. 2005;**99**:1802-1815

[20] Oswald-Mammosser M, Apprill M, Bachez P, et al. Pulmonary hemodynamics in chronic obstructive pulmonary disease of the emphysematous type. Respiration. 1991;**58**:304-310

[21] Montes de Oca M, Rassulo J, Celli BR. Respiratory muscle and cardiopulmonary function during exercise in very severe COPD. American Journal of Respiratory and Critical Care Medicine. 1996;**154**:1284-1289

[22] MacNee W. Pathophysiology of corpulmonale in chronic obstructive pulmonary disease: Part one. American Journal of Respiratory and Critical Care Medicine. 1994;**150**:833-852

[23] Kim HC, Mofarrahi M, Hussain NA. Skeletal muscle dysfunction in patients with chronic obstructive pulmonary disease. International Journal of COPD. 2008;**3**(4):637-658

[24] Creutzberg EC, Schols AM, Bothmer-Quaedvlieg FC, Wouters EF. Prevalence of an elevated resting energy expenditure in patients with chronic obstructive pulmonary disease in relation to body composition and lung function. European Journal of Clinical Nutrition. 1998;**52**:396-401

[25] Choudhury G, Rabinovich R, MacNee W. Comorbidities and systemic effects of chronic obstructive pulmonary disease. Clinics in Chest Medicine. 2014;**35**:101-130

[26] Schols AM, Broekhuizen R, Weling-Scheepers CA, Wouters EF. Body composition and mortality in chronic obstructive pulmonary disease. The American Journal of Clinical Nutrition. 2005;**82**:53-59

[27] Vermeeren MA, Creutzberg EC, Schols AM, et al. Prevalence of nutritional depletion in a large out-patient population of patients with COPD. Respiratory Medicine. 2006;**100**: 1349-1355

[28] Agusti AG. Systemic effects of chronic obstructive pulmonary disease. Proceedings of the American Thoracic Society. 2005;**2**:367-370 discussion 371-372

[29] Vermeeren MA, Wouters EF, Geraerts-Keeris AJ, Schols AM. Nutritional support in patients with chronic obstructive pulmonary disease during hospitalization for an acute exacerbation; a randomized controlled feasibility trial. Clinical Nutrition. 2004;**23**:1184-1192

[30] Brug J, Schols A, Mesters I. Dietary change, nutrition education and chronic obstructive pulmonary disease. Patient Education and Counseling. 2004;**52**:249-257

[31] Creutzberg EC, Wouters EF, Mostert R, et al. Efficacy of nutritional supplementation therapy in depleted patients with chronic obstructive pulmonary disease. Nutrition. 2003;**19**: 120-127

[32] Sehgal S, Dhooria S, Agarwal R. Chronic obstructive pulmonary disease and malnutrition in developing countries. Current Opinion in Pulmonary Medicine. 2017;**23**:139-148

[33] Hynninen KM, Breitve MH, Wiborg AB, et al. Psychological characteristics of patients with chronic obstructive pulmonary disease: A review. Journal of Psychosomatic Research. 2005;**59**:429-443

[34] Atlantis E, Fahey P, Cochrane B, et al. Bidirectional associations between clinically relevant depression or anxiety and COPD: A systematic review and meta-analysis. Chest. 2013;**144**:766-777

[35] Glassman AH, Helzer JE, Covey LS, et al. Smoking, smoking cessation, and major depression. JAMA. 1990;**264**:1546-1549

[36] Fergusson DM, Lynskey MT, Horwood LJ. Comorbidity between depressive disorders and nicotine dependence in a cohort of 16-year-olds. Archives of General Psychiatry. 1996; **53**:1043-1047

[37] Patton GC, Hibbert M, Rosier MJ, et al. Is smoking associated with depression and anxiety in teenagers? American Journal of Public Health. 1996;**86**:225-230

[38] Glassman AH, Covey LS, Stetner F, et al. Smoking cessation and the course of major depression: A follow-up study. Lancet. 2001;**357**:1929-1932

[39] Wiesbeck GA, Kuhl HC, Yaldizli O, et al. Tobacco smoking and depression--results from the WHO/ISBRA study. Neuropsychobiology. 2008;**57**:26-31

[40] Mineur YS, Picciotto MR. Nicotine receptors and depression: Revisiting and revising the cholinergic hypothesis. Trends in Pharmacological Sciences. 2010;**31**:580-586

[41] Sinden NJ, Stockley RA. Systemic inflammation and comorbidity in COPD: A result of 'overspill' of inflammatory mediators from the lungs? Review of the evidence. Thorax. 2010;**65**:930-936

[42] Eagan TM, Ueland T, Wagner PD, et al. Systemic inflammatory markers in COPD: Results from the Bergen COPD cohort study. The European Respiratory Journal. 2010;**35**:540-548

[43] Al-shair K, Kolsum U, Dockry R, et al. Biomarkers of systemic inflammation and depression and fatigue in moderate clinically stable COPD. Respiratory Research. 2011;**12**:3

[44] Marinho PE, Castro CM, Raposo MC, et al. Depressive symptoms, inflammatory markers and body composition in elderly with and without chronic obstructive pulmonary disease (COPD). Archives of Gerontology and Geriatrics. 2012;**54**:453-458

[45] van Dijk EJ, Vermeer SE, de Groot JC, et al. Arterial oxygen saturation, COPD, and cerebral small vessel disease. Journal of Neurology, Neurosurgery, and Psychiatry 2004;**75**:733-736.

[46] Campbell JJ 3rd, Coffey CE. Neuropsychiatric significance of subcortical hyperintensity. The Journal of Neuropsychiatry and Clinical Neurosciences. 2001;**13**:261-288

[47] Dunlop DD, Lyons JS, Manheim LM, et al. Arthritis and heart disease as risk factors for major depression: The role of functional limitation. Medical Care. 2004;**42**:502-511

[48] Penninx BW, van Tilburg T, Boeke AJ, et al. Effects of social support and personal coping resources on depressive symptoms: Different for various chronic diseases? Health Psychology 1998;**17**:551-558

[49] Emery CF, Leatherman NE, Burker EJ, MacIntyre NR. Psychological outcomes of a pulmonary rehabilitation program. Chest. 1991;**100**:613-617

[50] Emery CF, Schein RL, Hauck ER, MacIntyre NR. Psychological and cognitive outcomes of a randomized trial of exercise among patients with chronic obstructive pulmonary disease. Health Psychology. 1998;**17**:232-240

[51] O'Donnell DE, McGuire M, Samis L, Webb KA. The impact of exercise reconditioning on breathlessness in severe chronic airflow limitation. American Journal of Respiratory and Critical Care Medicine. 1995;**152**:2005-2013

[52] Garvey C, Bayles MP, Hamm LF, Hill K, Holland A, Limberg TM, Spruit MA. Pulmonary rehabilitation exercise prescription in chronic obstructive pulmonary disease: Review of selected guidelines. Journal of Cardiopulmonary Rehabilitation and Prevention. 2016;**36**: 75-83

[53] Mota S, Güell R, Barreiro E, Solanes I, Ramírez-Sarmiento A, OrozcoLevi M, et al. Clinical outcomes of expiratory muscle training in severe COPD patients. Respiratory Medicine. 2007;**101**(3):516-524

[54] Weiner P, McConnell A. Respiratory muscle training in chronic obstructive pulmonary disease: Inspiratory, expiratory, or both? Current Opinion in Pulmonary Medicine. 2005;**11**(2): 140-144

[55] Ramirez-Sarmiento A, Orozco-Levi M, Guell R, et al. Inspiratory muscle training in patients with chronic obstructive pulmonary disease: Structural adaptation and physiologic outcomes. American Journal of Respiratory and Critical Care Medicine. 2002;**166**(11):1491-1497

[56] Villafranca C, Borzone G, Leiva A, et al. Effect of inspiratory muscle training with an intermediate load on inspiratory power output in COPD. The European Respiratory Journal. 1998;**11**(1):28-33

[57] O'Donnell DE, Webb KA. Exertional breathlessness in patients with chronic airflow limitation. The American Review of Respiratory Disease. 1993;**148**(5):1351-1357

[58] Mador MJ, Deniz O, Aggarwal A, et al. Effect of respiratory muscle endurance training in patients with COPD undergoing pulmonary rehabilitation. Chest. 2005;**128**(3):1216-1224

[59] Larson JL, Covey MK, Wirtz SE, et al. Cycle ergometer and inspiratory muscle training in chronic obstructive pulmonary disease. American Journal of Respiratory and Critical Care Medicine. 1999;**160**(2):500-507

[60] Chen R, Li X, Guan N, Guo B, Wu W, Zhou Z, Huo Y, Chen X, Zhou L. Effectiveness of neuromuscular electrical stimulation for the rehabilitation of moderate-to-severe COPD: A meta-analysis. Intl J COPD. 2016;**11**:2965-2975

[61] Abdellaoui A, Préfaut C, Gouzi F, Couillard A, Coisy-Quivy M, Hugon G, Molinari N, Lafontaine T, Jonquet O, Laoudj-Chenivesse D, et al. Skeletal muscle effects of electrostimulation after COPD exacerbation: A pilot study. The European Respiratory Journal. 2011;**38**: 781-788

[62] Dal Corso S, Nápolis L, Malaguti C, Gimenes AC, Albuquerque A, Nogueira CR, De Fuccio MB, Pereira RD, Bulle A, McFarlane N, et al. Skeletal muscle structure and function in response to electrical stimulation in moderately impaired COPD patients. Respiratory Medicine. 2007;**101**:1236-1243

[63] McNamara RJ, McKeough ZJ, McKenzie DK, Alison JA. Water-based exercise in COPD with physical comorbidities: A randomised controlled trial. The European Respiratory Journal. 2013;**41**(6):1284-1291

[64] Leung RW, McKeough ZJ, Peters MJ, Alison JA. Short-form sun-style t'ai chi as an exercise training modality in people with COPD. The European Respiratory Journal. 2013;**41**(5): 1051-1057

[65] Yan JH, Guo YZ, Yao HM, Pan L. Effects of tai chi in patients with chronic obstructive pulmonary disease: Preliminary evidence. PLoS One. 2013;**8**(4) e61806

[66] Halbert RJ, Natoli JL, Gano A, Badamgarav E, Buist AS, Mannino DM. Global burden of COPD: Systematic review and meta-analysis. The European Respiratory Journal. 2006;**28**: 523-532

[67] Decramer M, Janssens W, Miravitlles M. Chronic obstructive pulmonary disease. Lancet. 2012;**379**:1341-1351

[68] McCarthy B, Casey D, Devane D, Murphy K, Murphy E, Lacasse Y. Pulmonary rehabilitation for chronic obstructive pulmonary disease (review). Cochrane Database of Systematic Reviews. 2015;(2). DOI: 10.1002/14651858.CD003793.pub3

[69] The Global Strategy for the Diagnosis, Management and Prevention of COPD, Global Initiative for Chronic Obstructive Lung Disease (GOLD) 2017. http://goldcopd.org.

[70] Evans RA, Singh SJ, Collier R, Williams JE, Morgan MD. Pulmonary rehabilitation is successful for COPD irrespective of MRC dyspnoea grade. Respiratory Medicine. 2009;**103**: 1070-1075

[71] Puente-Maestu L, Palange P, Casaburi R, Laveneziana P, Maltais F, Neder J, O'Donnell DE, Onorati P, Porszasz J, Rabinovich R, Rossiter HB, Singh S, Troosters T, Ward S. Use of exercise testing in the evaluation of interventional efficacy: An official ERS statement. The European Respiratory Journal. 2016;**47**:429-460

[72] Ringbaek T, Martinez G, Brøndum E, et al. Shuttle walking test as predictor of survival in chronic obstructive pulmonary disease patients enrolled in a rehabilitation program. Journal of Cardiopulmonary Rehabilitation and Prevention. 2010;**30**:409-414

[73] Steiner MC, Singh SJ, Morgan MD. The contribution of peripheral muscle function to shuttle walking performance in patients with chronic obstructive pulmonary disease. Journal of Cardiopulmonary Rehabilitation. 2005;**25**:43-49

[74] Lacasse Y, Wong E, Guyatt GH, et al. Meta-analysis of respiratory rehabilitation in chronic obstructive pulmonary disease. Lancet. 1996;**348**:1115-1119

[75] Wasserman K, Hansen JE, Sue DY, et al. Principles of Exercise Testing and Interpretation: Including Pathophysiology and Clinical Applications. 5th ed. Philadelphia: Lippincott Williams & Wilkins; 2011

[76] Puhan MA, Chandra D, Mosenifar Z, et al. The minimal important difference of exercise tests in severe COPD. The European Respiratory Journal. 2011;**37**:784-790

[77] Corhay JL, Nguyen D, Duysinx B, et al. Should we exclude elderly patients with chronic obstructive pulmonary disease from a long-time ambulatory pulmonary rehabilitation programme? Journal of Rehabilitation Medicine. 2012;**44**:466-472

[78] Troosters T, Casaburi R, Gosselink R, et al. Pulmonary rehabilitation in chronic obstructive pulmonary disease. American Journal of Respiratory and Critical Care Medicine. 2005;**172**:19-38

[79] Smid MSc E, Franssen F, Houben-Wilke S, Vanfleteren L, Janssen D, Wouters E, Spruit M. Responsiveness and MCID estimates for CAT, CCQ, and HADS in patients with COPD undergoing pulmonary rehabilitation: A prospective analysis. JAMDA. 2017;**18**:53e58

[80] Langer D. Rehabilitation in patients before and after lung transplantation. Respiration. 2015;**89**:353-362

[81] Wickerson L, Mathur S, Brooks D. Exercise training after lung transplantation: A systematic review. The Journal of Heart and Lung Transplantation. 2010;**29**:497-503

[82] Takaoka ST, Weinacker AB. The value of preoperative pulmonary rehabilitation. Thoracic Surgery Clinics. 2005;**15**:203-211

[83] Costache V, Chavanon O, St Raymond C, et al. Dramatic improvement in survival after lung transplantation over time: A single center experience. Transplantation Proceedings. 2009;**41**:687-691

[84] Troosters T, Demeyer H, Hornikx M, et al. Pulmonary rehabilitation. Clinics in Chest Medicine. 2014;**35**:241-249

[85] Van der Woude BT, Kropmans TJB, Douma KW, et al. Peripheral muscle force and exercise capacity in lung transplant candidates. International Journal of Rehabilitation Research. 2002;**25**:351-355

[86] Mathur S, Reid WD, Levy RD. Exercise limitation in recipients of lung transplants. Physical Therapy. 2004;**84**:1178-1187

[87] Wang XN, Williams TJ, McKenna MJ, Li JL, Fraser SF, Side EA, et al. Skeletal muscle oxidative capacity, fiber type, and metabolites after lung transplantation. American Journal of Respiratory and Critical Care Medicine. 1999;**160**(1):57

[88] Krieger AC, Szidon P, Kesten S. Skeletal muscle dysfunction in lung transplantation. The Journal of Heart and Lung Transplantation. 2000;**19**:392-400

[89] Pantoja JG, Andrade FH, Stokic DS, Frost AE, Eschenbacher WL, Reid MB. Respiratory and limb muscle function in lung allograft recipients. American Journal of Respiratory and Critical Care Medicine. 1999;**160**:1205-1211

[90] Williams TJ, Patterson GA, McClean PA, Zamel N, Maurer JR. Maximal exercise testing in single and double lung transplant recipients. The American Review of Respiratory Disease. 1992;**145**(1):101-105

[91] Lands LC, Smountas AA, Mesiano G, Brosseau L, Shennib H, Charbonneau M, Gauthier R. Maximal exercise capacity and peripheral skeletal muscle function following lung transplantation. The Journal of Heart and Lung Transplantation. 1999;**18**(2):113-120

[92] Schuurmans MM, Benden C, Inci I. Practical approach to early postoperative management of lung transplant recipients. Swiss Medical Weekly. 2013;**143**:137-173

[93] Downs AM. Physical therapy in lung transplantation. Physical Therapy. 1996;**76**(6): 626-642

[94] National Emphysema Treatment Trial Group. A randomized trial comparing lung volume-reduction surgery with medical therapy for severe emphysema. The New England Journal of Medicine. 2003;**348**(21):2059-2073

[95] Pompeo E, Marino M, Nofroni I, Matteucci G, Mineo TC. Reduction pneumoplasty versus respiratory rehabilitation in severe emphyse- ma: A randomized study. The Annals of Thoracic Surgery. 2000;**70**(3):948-954

[96] Criner GJ, Cordova FC, Furukawa S, Kuzma AM, Travaline JM, Leyenson V, O'Brien GM. Prospective randomized trial comparing bilateral lung volume reduction surgery to pulmonary rehabilitation in severe chronic obstructive pulmonary disease. American Journal of Respiratory and Critical Care Medicine. 1999;**160**(6):2018-2027

[97] Koegelenberg CF, Theron J, Dheda K, Bruwer JW, Allwood BW, Vorster J, Groote-Bidlingmaier F, Slebos DJ, Shah PL, Herth FJF. Recommendations for the use of endoscopic lung volume reduction in South Africa: Role in the treatment of emphysema. SAMJ. 2015;**105**:810-815

[98] Gao K, PM Y, JH S, He CQ, Liu LX, Zhou YB, Pu Q, Che GW. Cardiopulmonary exercise testing screening and pre-operative pulmonary rehabilitation reduce postoperative complications and improve fast-track recovery after lung cancer surgery: A study for 342 cases. Thorac Cancer. 2015 Jul;**6**(4):443-449

[99] Adamsen L, Midtgaard J, Andersen C, Quist M, Moeller T, Roerth M. Transforming the nature of fatigue through exercise: Qualitative findings from a multidimensional exercise programme in cancer patients undergoing chemotherapy. European Journal of Cancer Care. 2004;**13**(4):362-370

[100] Pasqua F, D'Angelillo R, Mattei F, et al. Pulmonary rehabilitation following radical chemoradiation in locally advanced non surgical NSCLC: Preliminary evidences. Lung Cancer. 2012;**76**(2):258-259

[101] Tarumi S, Yokomise H, Gotoh M, et al. Pulmonary rehabilitation during induction chemoradiotherapy for lung cancer improves pulmonary function. Journal of Thoracic and Cardiovascular Surgery. 2015;**149**(2):569-573

[102] Keays KS, Harris SR, Lucyshyn JM, MacIntyre DL. Effects of pilates exercises on shoulder range of motion, pain, mood, and upper extremity function in women living with breast cancer: A pilot study. Physical Therapy. 2008;**88**(4):494-510

[103] Clay CA, Perera S, Wagner JM, Miller ME, Nelson JB, Grrenspan SL. Physical function in men with prostate cancer on androgen deprivation therapy. Physical Therapy. 2007;**87**(10):1325-1333

[104] Bicego D, Brown K, Ruddick M, Storey D, Wong C, Harris SR. Exercise for women with or at risk for breast cancer-related lymphedema. Physical Therapy. 2006;**86**(10):1398-13405

[105] Albrecht TA, Taylor AG. Physical activity in patients with advanced-stage cancer: A systematic review of the literature. Clinical Journal of Oncology Nursing. 2012;**16**(3):293-300

[106] Bolton CE, Bevan- Smith EF, Blakey JD, et al. British Thoracic Society guideline on pulmonary rehabilitation in adults. Thorax. 2013;**68**:1-30

[107] Puhan M, Scharplatz M, Troosters T, Walters EH, Steurer J. Pulmonary rehabilitation following exacerbations of chronic obstructive pulmonary disease. Cochrane Database of Systematic Reviews. 2011;**1**:5305

[108] Lacasse Y, Goldstein R, Lasserson TJ, Martin S. Pulmonary rehabilitation for chronic obstructive pulmonary disease. Cochrane Database of Systematic Reviews. 2006;**4**:37-93

[109] Wedzicha JA, Miravitlles M, Hurst JR, Calverley P, Albert K, Anzueto A, Criner J, Papi A, Rabe KF, Rigau D, Sliwinski P, Tonia T, Vestbo J, Wilson KC, Krishnan JA. Management of COPD exacerbations: A European Respiratory Society/American Thoracic Society guideline. The European Respiratory Journal. 2017;**49**:1600791

[110] Ntoumenopoulos G. Rehabilitation during mechanical ventilation: Review of the recent literature. Intensive & Critical Care Nursing. 2015;**31**(3):125-132

[111] Sommers J, Engelbert RHH, Dettling-Ihnenfeldt D, Gosselink R, Spronk PE, Nollet F, van der Schaaf M. Physiotherapy in the intensive care unit: An evidence-based, expert driven, practical statement and rehabilitation recommendations. Clinical Rehabilitation 2015;**29**(11):1051-1063

[112] Nydahl P, Sricharoenchai T, Chandra S, Kundt FS, Huang M, Fischill M, Needham DM. Safety of patient mobilization and rehabilitation in the intensive care unit. Systematic review with meta-analysis. Annals of the American Thoracic Society. 2017 May;**14**(5): 766-777

[113] Hoff J, Tjonna AE, Steinshamn S, et al. Maximal strength training of the legs in COPD: A therapy for mechanical inefficiency. Medicine and Science in Sports and Exercise. 2007;**39**: 220-226

[114] Menadue C, Piper AJ, van 't Hul AJ, Wong KK. Non-invasive ventilation during exercise training for people with chronic obstructive pulmonary disease (review). Cochrane Data base of Systematic Reviews. 2014(5). Art. No.: CD007714

[115] Garrod R, Mikelsons C, Paul EA, Wedzicha JA. Randomized controlled trial of domiciliary noninvasive positive pressure ventilation and physical training in severe chronic obstructive pulmonary disease. American Journal of Respiratory and Critical Care Medicine. 2000;**162**:1335-1341

[116] Hornikx M, Van Remoortel H, Demeyer H, et al. The influence of comorbidities on outcomes of pulmonary rehabilitation pro- grams in patients with COPD: A systematic review. BioMed Research International. 2013;**2013**:146-148

[117] Carreiro A, Santos J, Rodrigues F. Impact of comorbidities in pulmonary rehabilitation outcomes in patients with chronic obstructive pulmonary disease. Revista Portuguesa de Pneumologia. 2013;**19**(3):106-113

[118] Crisafulli E, Costi S, Luppi F, et al. Role of comorbidities in a cohort of patients with COPD undergoing pulmonary rehabilitation. Thorax. 2008;**63**:487-492

[119] Crisafulli E, Gorgone P, Vagaggini B, et al. Efficacy of standard rehabilitation in COPD outpatients with comorbidities. European Respiratory Journal. 2010;**36**:1042-1048

[120] Walsh JR, McKeough ZJ, Morris NR, et al. Metabolic disease and participant age are independent predictors of response to pulmonary rehabilitation. Journal of Cardiopulmonary Rehabilitation and Prevention. 2013;**33**:249-256

[121] McNamara RJ, McKeough ZJ, McKenzie DK, Alison JA. Water- based exercise in COPD with physical comorbidities: A ran- domised controlled trial. European Respiratory Journal. 2013;**41**:1284-1291

[122] Tunsupon P, Lal A, Khamis MA, Mador MJ. Comorbidities in patients with chronic obstructive pulmonary disease and pulmonary rehabilitation outcomes. Journal of Cardiopulmonary Rehabilitation and Prevention. 2017;**00**:1-9

[123] Emery CF, Shermer RL, Hauck ER, Hsiao ET, MacIntyre NR. Cognitive and psychological outcomes of exercise in a 1-year follow-up study of patients with chronic obstructive pulmonary disease. Health Psychology. 2003;**22**(6):598-604

[124] Corhay J, Dang DN, Cauwenberge H, Louis R. Pulmonary rehabilitation and COPD: Providing patients a good environment for optimizing therapy. International Journal of COPD. 2014;**9**:27-39

[125] Rochester CL, Vogiatzis I, Holland AE, Lareau SC, Marciniuk DD, Puhan MA, et al. An official American Thoracic Society/European Respiratory Society policy statement: Enhancing implementation, use, and delivery of pulmonary rehabilitation. American Journal of Respiratory and Critical Care Medicine. 2015;**192**(11):1373-1386

[126] Vasilopoulou M, Papaioannou AI, Kaltsakas G, et al. Home-based maintenance tele-rehabilitation reduces the risk for acute exacerbations of COPD, hospitalisations and emergency department visits. The European Respiratory Journal. 2017;**49**:1602129